In-patient Physiotherapy

Management of Or

D1336360

Acquisitions editor: Heidi Allen
Development editor: Myriam Brearley
Production controller: Anthony Read
Desk editor: Jane Campbell
Cover designer: Helen Brockway

In-patient Physiotherapy

Management of Orthopaedic Surgery

Lucy S Chipchase
MAPA, MAppSc(Physiotherapy)
Lecturer and 2nd Year Coordinator

School of Physiotherapy
University of South Australia
North Terrace
Adelaide SA 5000, Australia
lucy.chipchase@unisa.edu.au

and

Scott A Brumby
BM, BS, PhD, FRACS(Orth)
Orthopaedic Surgeon, Wakefield Orthopaedic Clinic
Visiting Orthopaedic Surgeon, Royal Adelaide Hospital
Lecturer, Department of Orthopaedics and Trauma, University of Adelaide

Wakefield Orthopaedic Clinic
270 Wakefield Street
Adelaide SA 5000, Australia
scottbrumby@woc.com.au

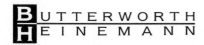

BUTTERWORTH
HEINEMANN

OXFORD AUCKLAND BOSTON JOHANNESBURG MELBOURNE NEW DELHI

Butterworth-Heinemann
Linacre House, Jordan Hill, Oxford OX2 8DP
225 Wildwood Avenue, Woburn, MA 01801-2041
A division of Reed Educational and Professional Publishing Ltd

℞ A member of the Reed Elsevier plc group

First published 2001

British Library Cataloguing in Publication Data
Chipchase, Lucy S.
   In-patient physiotherapy: management of orthopaedic surgery
   1.   Physical therapy   2.   Orthopedic surgery
   I.   Title   II.   Brumby, Scott A.
   616.7′062

Library of Congress Cataloguing in Publication Data
A catalogue record for this book is available from the Library of Congress

ISBN 0 7506 4459 1

Typeset by Keyword Typesetting Services Ltd, Wallington, Surrey
Printed and bound by MPG Books Ltd, Bodmin, Cornwall

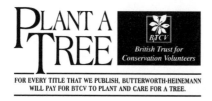

Contents

Foreword   vii

Preface   ix

Acknowledgements   xi

Abbreviations   xiii

Chapter 1   Principles of orthopaedic surgery   1

**Chapter 2   Medical investigations, equipment and
              common medication   26**

**Chapter 3   Principles of physiotherapy assessment
              and management   35**

Chapter 4   Gait and mobility education   51

Chapter 5   Transfer and lifting techniques   66

Chapter 6   Hip surgery   78

Chapter 7   Knee surgery   102

Chapter 8   Shoulder surgery   124

Chapter 9   Surgery of the foot and ankle   146

Index   153

Foreword

Physiotherapy management of patients following orthopaedic surgery or trauma represents one of the major contributions which physiotherapists make to patient care. A key component of the preparation of physiotherapy students as beginning practitioners is that component which is spent in acquiring the knowledge base, the clinical reasoning skills, assessment and treatment skills to manage orthopaedic patients post surgical intervention.

This text is primarily written for undergraduate physiotherapy students preparing for, and/or undertaking an in-patient orthopaedic clinical placement for the first time. It will also be of excellent value for junior physiotherapists who have not had prior opportunity to work in an in-patient orthopaedic setting, and for physiotherapists wishing to re-enter the workforce in an in-patient orthopaedic setting after a period out of practice.

This text, written by an experienced orthopaedic physiotherapist and a consultant orthopaedic surgeon, fills a gap between medical orthopaedic texts and those concerned with orthopaedic physiotherapy management in the outpatient setting. There are few texts which cover the essential physiotherapy management of common orthopaedic surgical conditions of a non-spinal nature in as clear and concise a way as does this book.

The book provides a step-by-step introduction to the more common orthopaedic surgical procedures in the hip, knee, shoulder, foot and ankle regions and their physiotherapy management. Early chapters outline the principles of orthopaedic surgery and the principles of physiotherapy assessment and management. Generic skills for gait and mobility education, and for transfer and lifting of patients are clearly and concisely described. A chapter on medical investigations, common medications and equipment also precedes the chapters devoted to hip, knee, shoulder, foot and ankle surgery and their management.

With its very practical approach, this book will be invaluable in providing physiotherapy students and junior physiotherapists with the skills necessary for the management of patients post orthopaedic surgery.

Professor Ruth Grant
Professor of Physiotherapy
Pro Vice Chancellor
Division of Health Sciences
University of South Australia

Preface

This book has been written as an introduction to clinical physiotherapy from admission to discharge of the most common orthopaedic surgical procedures. The intention is to provide undergraduate students with sufficient information before a clinical placement to an orthopaedic ward.

In-patient rehabilitation protocols and exercises are provided for some surgical procedures. These are guidelines of the most commonly prescribed exercises. The inclusion of common exercises and protocols is not meant to replace the need for clinical reasoning and problem solving, but to provide a base from which students can further develop and learn.

Acknowledgements

Lucy Chipchase would like to thank the staff at the School of Physiotherapy, University of South Australia, for their encouragement and support to write this book, particularly Frances Blaney, Karen Grimmer, Andrea Warden-Flood and Marie Williams. Thanks also to Sonia Russo, Rosey Boehm, David Wilson and Cheryl Buck for helping with the photographs and to Anne McIntosh from Smith and Nephew for access to surgical components and rehabilitation equipment. Finally, special thanks to Patricia Murphy and Penny Munro for their friendship, support and belief.

Scott Brumby would like to thank his wife Jodi and daughter Isabella Ruby for their support and understanding whilst writing this book.

Abbreviations

Abd	Abduction
Add	Adduction
ACL	Anterior cruciate ligament
ADL	Activities of daily living
AE	Above elbow
A/E	Accident and emergency
AFO	Ankle foot orthosis
AK	Above knee
AMBRI	Atraumatic multidirectional often bilateral most requiring rehabilitation and if requires surgery, then treated with an inferior capsular shift
AMP	Austin–Moore prosthesis
AO	Arbeitsgemeinschaft für Osteosynthesefragen
A-P	Antero-posterior
AROM	Active range of movement
AVN	Avascular necrosis (better known as osteonecrosis)
BD	Twice daily
BE	Below elbow
BK	Below knee
BMP	Bone morphogenic protein
BP	Blood pressure
CBE	Complete blood examination (Hb, WCC and platelet count)
CBP	Complete blood picture (interchangeable with CBE)
CC	Calcaneo-cuboid
CKC	Closed kinetic chain
CMC	Carpo-metacarpal
CNS	Central nervous system
CPM	Continuous passive motion
CR	Closed reduction
CRP	C-reactive protein
CSF	Cerebrospinal fluid
CT	Computerized tomography
CVS	Cardiovascular system
CWMS	Colour, warmth, movement, sensation
CXR	Chest X-ray
Daily	Once daily
DB&C	Deep breath and cough exercises

D/C	Discharge
DCP	Dynamic compression plate
DCS	Dynamic condylar screw
DEXA	Dual energy X-ray absorptimetry
DHS	Dynamic hip screw
DIP	Distal interphalangeal
DPC	Delayed primary closure
DSU	Day Surgery Unit
DVT	Deep veined thrombosis
E	Extension
ECG	Electrocardiogram
EF	External fixation
E/O	Excision of
ESR	Erythrocyte sedimentation rate
EUA	Examination under anaesthesia
F	Flexion
F&A	Foot and ankle exercises
FH	Family history
FRC	Functional residual capacity
FWB	Full weight bearing
GA	General anaesthetic
GH	General health
GIT	Gastro-intestinal system
HA	Heavy assist
Hb	Haemoglobin
HRT	Hormone replacement therapy
HV	Hallux valgus
IV	Intravenous
ICU	Intensive Care Unit
IDC	In-dwelling catheter
IF	Internal fixation
IM	Intramuscular
IM	Intramedullary
INR	International normalized ratio
IP	Interphalangeal
IRQ	Inner range quadriceps exercises
ISQ	Condition unaltered (in status quo)
IVT	Intravenous therapy
KAFO	Knee–ankle–foot orthosis
K-wire	Kirschner wire
LA	Local anaesthetic
LA	Light assist
LCPD	Legg–Calve–Perthes disease
LFT	Liver function test
LHB	Long head of biceps
MA	Moderate assist
mane	In the morning
MBA	Multiple biochemical analysis
MBA	Motor bike accident
MCL	Medial collateral ligament

MCP	Metacarpophalangeal
MRI	Magnetic resonance imaging
MSS	Musculoskeletal system
MT	Metatarsal
MTP	Metatarsophalangeal joint
MUA	Manipulation under anaesthesia
MVA	Motor vehicle accident
nocté	At night
NOF	Neck of femur
NSAID	Non-steroidal anti-inflammatory drug
NWB	Non-weight bearing
OA	Osteoarthritis
O/A	On arrival/admission
O/E	On examination
OKC	Open kinetic chain
OOP	Out of plaster
OPD	Out-patient department
OR	Open reduction
ORIF	Open reduction internal fixation
PAC	Pressure area care
PC	Present complaint (present condition)
PCA	Patient-controlled analgesia
PCL	Posterior cruciate ligament
PE	Pulmonary embolus
PH	Past history
PIP	Proximal interphalangeal
PMMA	Poly-methyl-methacrylate
PO	Orally
POMR	Problem-oriented medical record
POP	Plaster of Paris
PRN	As occasion arises (as required)
PROM	Passive range of movement
PTB	Patellar tendon bearing
PWB	Partial weight bearing
QID	Four times daily
RA	Rheumatoid arthritis
RIB	Rest in bed
R/O	Removal of
ROM	Range of movement
ROS	Removal of sutures or review of systems
ROP	Removal of plaster
RS	Respiratory system
Rx	Treatment
SA	Standby assistance
SB	Standby
S/B	Seen by
SCFE	Slipped capital femoral epiphysis
SF-36	Short form 36
SG	Static gluteal exercises
SH	Social history

SLR	Straight leg raise
SOB	Shortness of breath
SOBOE	Shortness of breath on exertion
SOOB	Sit out of bed
SQ	Static quadriceps exercises
T	One tablet
TDS	Three times daily
THR (THA)	Total hip replacement (arthroplasty)
TKR (TKA)	Total knee replacement (arthroplasty)
TN	Talo-navicular
TPR	Temperature, pulse, respiration
TPT	Total plaster time
TSD	To see doctor
TSR (TSA)	Total shoulder replacement (arthroplasty)
TT	Two tablets
TTWB	Toe-touch weight bearing
TUBS	Traumatic unidirectional associated with a Bankart lesion requiring surgery
UTI	Urinary tract infection
VMO	Vastus medialis oblique
WBAT	Weight bearing as tolerated
WBC	White blood count
WCC	White cell count
XR	X-ray

Other Definitions

#	Fracture
5% D	Five per cent dextrose
4% D and 1/5th N/S	Four per cent dextrose and 1/5th normal saline
Hartmann's	Balanced electrolyte solution
KCl	Potassium chloride
N/S	Normal saline

CHAPTER 1

Principles of orthopaedic surgery

This chapter will outline the basic science of bone and soft tissue healing, common orthopaedic disease processes, classification and basic surgical management of fractures and major musculoskeletal trauma.

Basic science of bone and soft tissues

Bone

Bone consists of cells, type I collagen, several non-collagenous proteins, small amounts of other molecules and calcium hydroxyapatite crystals. There are three main types of bone cells, osteoblasts, osteocytes and osteoclasts. All three types of bone cell originate from the same progenitor cell. Osteoblasts form the type I collagen that is required by bone and are responsive to various chemical mediators that influence bone formation. Osteocytes are osteoblasts that have been surrounded by mineralized bone matrix and are important in calcium regulation and bone remodelling. Osteoclasts are large multi-nucleated cells that resorb bone.

There are two histological types of bone. Woven bone is the primitive bone that is found in the embryo, newborn, fracture callus, the metaphysis of growing bones, some tumours, osteogenesis imperfecta and in Paget's disease. Lamellar or mature bone first appears 1 month after birth and by age four most normal bone is lamellar, remodelled woven bone. Stress-orientated collagen gives lamellar bone its specific biomechanical properties.

Bone is also described as either trabecular or cortical. Trabecular bone is found in the metaphysis and epiphysis of long bones and in cuboid type bones such as the vertebrae. It consists of a network of connecting plates and rods, with a 50–90 per cent porosity, and it is predominately compression loaded. Cortical bone is found in the diaphysis of long bones and the envelope of cuboid bones. It is a solid containing a series of voids, with less than 30 per cent porosity, that is subject to compression, bending and torsional forces. Bone is stronger in compression than tension.

Tendons

Tendons consist of type I collagen, proteoglycan matrix and fibroblasts. They have a complex structure with five collagen molecules forming a microfibril that are arranged to form sub-fibrils and fibrils. Fibrils are incorporated with proteoglycans, glycoproteins, fibroblasts and water to form fascicles. Fascicles are bound by loose connective tissue (endotenon), blood vessels, lymphatics and nerves to form tendons. The epitenon is the layer that covers the surface of a tendon. The paratenon is the sheath that covers tendons that are not enclosed in a synovial sheath. The mesotenon is the sheath that in-folds over tendons inside synovial sheaths. The blood supply is from the perimysium, periosteal insertion and vessels in the para- or mesotenon.

Tendons that have a paratenon cover heal with a vascular repair. The defect fills with fibrin clot and inflammatory products, then undifferentiated fibroblasts and capillaries. Collagen initially is formed perpendicular to the long axis of the tendon, and by 3–4 week orientates with the long axis of the tendon (secondary remodelling) with reduced scar formation and increased tensile strength. At 20 weeks the histology is normal. Tendons that have a mesotenon cover heal with an avascular repair. There is intrinsic healing from the tendon if motion is allowed and granulation from the tendon sheath if immobilized.

Ligaments

Ligaments consist of type I collagen, elastin, proteoglycan matrix and fibroblasts. The structure is similar to tendons and they insert into bone by a specialized transition of fibrocartilage or directly into the periosteum. Ligaments have less collagen which is less organized than tendons and have more matrix. Ligaments have a microvascular supply from the insertion site and specialized nerve endings for pain and proprioception.

Ligament injuries can be graded I to III. A grade I injury is caused by overstretching without disruption resulting in micro-haemorrhages. In a grade II injury the continuity of the tendon is maintained but there may be tears and haemorrhage. In grade III injuries there is complete disruption of the ligament. Healing is that of a vascular tissue with stages of fibrin clot, inflammation, organization, vascularization, proliferation, matrix formation and remodelling. Type III and type I collagen is formed initially then mainly type I later. Collagen organization and orientation occurs after 6 weeks and is normal after 12 months. In most cases surgical repair is not required and healing is enhanced by gentle range of motion and prevention of instability with splintage.

Meniscus

The meniscus of the knee consists of fibrocartilage which is comprised of type I collagen orientated circumferentially with some radial fibres, biphasic matrix of proteoglycans, glycoproteins and water, and fibrochondrocyte cells. The role of the meniscus is for load distribution, shock absorption, joint lubrication and as a secondary stabilizer of the knee.

The menisci transmit 50–90 per cent of the knee joint force and loading results in radial centrifugal forces that are resisted by anterior and posterior attachments of the menisci.

The blood supply is from the peripheral peri-meniscal plexus that only penetrates the outer 10–30 per cent. Peripheral vascular tears in the outer 10–30 per cent can initiate a healing response and can be repaired with meniscal sutures. Tears in the inner 70 per cent will not heal and should be resected.

Articular cartilage

Cartilage consists of proteoglycans, type II collagen (also small amounts of type V, VI, IX, X, XI), water, glycoproteins, chondrocytes and other minor components that probably have an important, but as yet undefined role. There is no nerve supply or blood vessels and cartilage has a reduced immune response.

Proteoglycans hold the collagen network apart and decrease tissue permeability, therefore holding water. The high hydrostatic pressure allows cartilage to support load and reduces stress on cartilage matrix. Motion and load are required to maintain normal cartilage.

Superficial lacerations will not heal if the laceration does not cross the deep calcified layer as there is no stimulus to healing. Chondrocytes may proliferate nearby and form matrix but they do not migrate into the lesion. Deep lacerations will disrupt the underlying subchondral bone resulting in fibrin clot formation whilst inflammatory cells migrate and proliferate. The repair tissue formed is a mix of hyaline cartilage, fibrocartilage and fibrous tissue, and is a biomechanically inferior tissue. Blunt impact can damage the cartilage by single high loads or by multiple impact. High impact may lead to shearing of the cartilage from the subchondral bone and may stiffen the cartilage–bone interface and thin the cartilage, resulting in osteoarthritis.

Common disease processes

Osteoarthritis

Osteoarthritis is a slowly progressive monoarticular or, less commonly, polyarticular disorder of unknown aetiology and obscure pathogenesis. It is more common with increased age but is not a natural consequence. It may be described as a primary disorder or secondary due to joint incongruity, sequelae of other diseases, joint and ligament laxity, Paget's disease and inflammatory arthropathies.

The pathology of osteoarthritis involves fissuring and local erosive changes in articular cartilage, cartilage loss and destruction, subchondral sclerosis, cyst formation and osteophyte formation. The joint capsule becomes thickened, there is an inflammatory infiltrate of the synovium and capsule and bone is remodelled with thickened cortices and changes in trabeculae stress lines. Articular cartilage has reduced proteoglycan, increased water content and the collagen is less ordered.

Cartilage degeneration is commonly graded as

Grade 1   Softening of articular cartilage
Grade 2   Fibrillation and fissuring of articular cartilage
Grade 3   Partial thickness cartilage loss, clefts and chondral flaps
Grade 4   Full thickness cartilage loss with bone exposed.

Osteoarthritis results in an intermittent disability with pain often worse on rising from bed and at the end of the day, aggravated by activity and exaggerated by extremes of movement. Radiographs show joint space narrowing, sub-articular sclerosis, bone cysts and osteophytes. Bone density is either normal or increased. There may be evidence of other pathology such as previous trauma, congenital deformities or chondrocalcinosis.

Rheumatoid arthritis

Rheumatoid arthritis is a chronic, systemic, inflammatory disorder of unknown aetiology resulting in a symmetrical polyarthropathy, initially involving the small joints with a variety of extra-articular manifestations. It affects 3 per cent of the population and usually presents in females during the 3–4th decade of life. Radiographs initially show local osteoporosis adjacent to the joints followed by marginal erosions and joint space narrowing (Fig. 1.1). The end result is destruction and deformity. Blood markers such as the ESR (erythrocyte sedimentation rate) and CRP (C-reactive protein) are often raised and rheumatoid factor can be found in the blood in 80 per cent of people with rheumatoid arthritis.

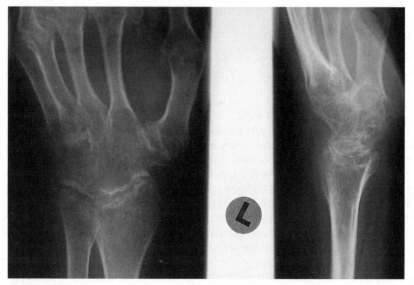

Figure 1.1. Antero-posterior and lateral radiographs of the wrist and hand of a patient with rheumatoid arthritis.

Treatment is directed towards arresting the synovitis with rest, splints, non-steroidal anti-inflammatory drugs (NSAIDs), steroids, specific anti-rheumatoid drugs and synovectomy, in some cases, where medical management has failed. Efforts are made to prevent deformity with physiotherapy, splints and possibly tendon reconstruction and stabilization. Reconstruction may be required with arthrodesis (fusion of the joint), excision arthroplasty or joint replacement. Rehabilitation is enhanced with functional aids and home modification.

Osteonecrosis

Defined as death of bone from a lack of blood supply, often called avascular necrosis. The peak incidence is between age 40 and 50 years. The most common sites are the proximal femur, distal femur (medial femoral condyle), proximal humerus, talus, lunate, capitulum and the metatarsal heads. The aetiology includes trauma with interruption to the local blood supply, steroid use, alcohol abuse, idiopathic, and several less common disorders including infection, post-irradiation and sickle cell disease.

The clinical features are pain, stiffness and commonly severe night pain. Radiographic changes vary with the course of the disease and may initially be normal. Later they demonstrate increased density from compression of the trabeculae, collapse and new bone formation on dead trabeculae, subchondral fracture and later degenerate changes. Bone scans and magnetic resonance imaging (MRI) may be used to assist with the diagnosis.

Osteoporosis

Osteoporosis is a bone disorder characterized by a decreased bone mass and an increased risk of fracture. The bone composition is normal but bone per unit volume is less than the 95th percentile of normal values. Osteoporosis affects one in three women in Australia with 5–10 per cent having osteoporotic crush fractures by age 60 and 40 per cent by age 80. Aetiology includes oestrogen withdrawal (post-menopause, post-surgical), impaired metabolism, long-term calcium deficiency, secondary hyperparathyroidism, inactivity, genetic factors, smoking and alcohol.

Thirty per cent of bone mass must be lost before it can be detected on routine plain X-ray. Therefore bone density measurements are made with special imaging called DEXA scans (dual energy X-ray absorptimetry). Treatment is guided by a ratio of the calculated bone density with normal values from healthy young adults and age-matched controls. Treatment is directed to correcting the underlying cause (diet, smoking, alcohol, exercise). Medical treatment can be directed using published guidelines and includes HRT (hormone replacement therapy), calcium supplements, biphosphonates (medications that regulate bone turnover), anabolic steroids, fluoride and calcitonin.

Paget's disease

This condition is characterized by high rates of bone resorption and disorganized immature new bone formation resulting in abnormal remodelling of bone. It affects 3 per cent of the population over 40 years of age. The primary abnormality is thought to lie in the osteoclasts but the precise cause remains unknown. Paget's disease is caused by infection with a common and widespread virus superimposed on genetic variation for susceptibility and perhaps severity of disease.

Paget's disease presents with a variable picture with the majority being discovered incidentally following X-ray or elevated alkaline phosphatase. Only a minority of patients become symptomatic (5 per cent).

Most patients require no treatment. Non-steroidal anti-inflammatories and analgesics useful. Patients with symptomatic disease are usually treated with calcitonin or biphosphonates. Complications include pathological fractures, sarcomatous change, nerve compression resulting in pain, blindness or deafness, spinal canal stenosis, arthritis of joints affected with Paget's (hip or knee) but only if sub-articular bone is involved (bone either soft or brittle) and high output cardiac failure due to prolonged increased bone blood flow. There is a slightly higher incidence of aseptic loosening of joint implants than in primary osteoarthritis (15–17 per cent before 10 years).

Orthopaedic trauma

Definitions

Fracture	A break in the continuity of a bone that may be complete or incomplete.
Joint dislocation	The joint surfaces are completely displaced and the articular surfaces are no longer in contact. With severe trauma, a fracture and dislocation may occur at the same time. This commonly occurs in the ankle (Fig. 1.2).
Joint subluxation	A lesser degree of joint displacement such that the articular surfaces are still partly apposed.

Traumatic fractures

These fractures are perhaps the most common type of fracture and are caused by the application of a sudden and extreme force. The direction of the force generally results in predictable fracture patterns. This force may be direct or indirect. In conjunction with bone damage there will often be associated damage to the soft tissues, such as surrounding muscles, nerves and ligaments.

Direct trauma results in the fracture occurring at the point of impact and is usually associated with soft tissue injury, e.g. falling from a ladder and landing on both feet commonly causes bilateral fractured calcaneum. Whereas indirect trauma results in a fracture away from the point of

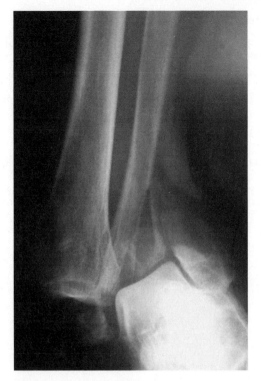

Figure 1.2. Fracture dislocation of the ankle
joint.

impact, e.g. the lower leg caught in a hole in the ground sustaining a
twisting force may cause a spiral fracture of the fibula. These fractures
are not as commonly associated with soft tissue injury.

Pathological fractures

These fractures occur spontaneously with no known force or trivial
trauma to a bone that has already been weakened by disease. Diseases
that may weaken the bone structure include metastatic tumour (prostate,
breast, thyroid, lung), primary bone tumour, osteoporosis and other metabolic bone diseases.

Stress fractures

Stress fractures are caused by activity that results in repeated stress or
force being applied to the bone. This repetitive activity may lead to weakening of the bone. With a few exceptions, stress fractures most commonly
occur in the bones of the lower limb especially the metatarsals, tibia and
fibula.

Avulsion fractures

Avulsion fractures arise when a sudden extreme muscular contraction results in detachment of the segment of bone to which the tendon and muscle is attached. Ligaments may also be tractioned sufficiently to break off the bony attachment site, as seen around the distal fibula.

Fracture classification

There is a myriad of classification schemes for fractures. In simple terms fractures can be described in the terms of the location, the degree of displacement, the shape and whether it extends into a joint.

Location

In the long bones a fracture can be described as proximal, mid-shaft or distal (Fig. 1.3), whilst fractures of the spine are described according to the vertebrae involved, e.g. third lumbar vertebra.

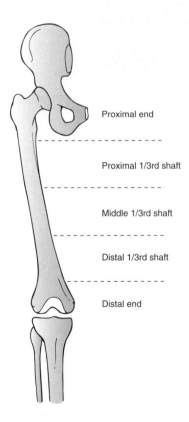

Proximal end

Proximal 1/3rd shaft

Middle 1/3rd shaft

Distal 1/3rd shaft

Distal end

Figure 1.3. Area of fracture in long bone.

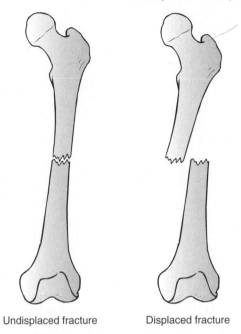

Undisplaced fracture   Displaced fracture

Figure 1.4. Undisplaced and displaced fracture.

Degree of displacement

Displaced

Where the fracture segments may override each other, are lateral to each other or extremely distracted from each other (Fig. 1.4).

Undisplaced

The fracture ends are in alignment (Fig. 1.4).

Open or closed

Open

The fractures or force causing the fracture has resulted in the skin being breached (Fig. 1.5). The skin may be broken outside (from the force) or from within where the bone end pushes through the soft tissue. These fractures are more susceptible to infection. In the past these were called compound fractures.

Closed

The skin remains intact (Fig. 1.5). Previously known as simple fractures.

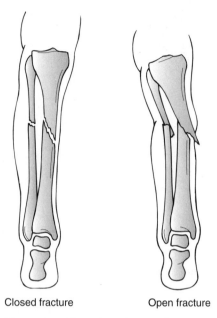

Closed fracture   Open fracture

Figure 1.5. Closed and open fracture of the tibia and fibula.

Shape or line of the fracture

A variety of different shapes or patterns of fractures can occur depending on the force applied to sustain the fracture (Fig. 1.6). Most common shapes are:

Transverse

Directly across the bone.

Oblique

Diagonal fracture line.

Spiral

Around the bone.

Comminuted

Having three or more fragments (Fig. 1.7).

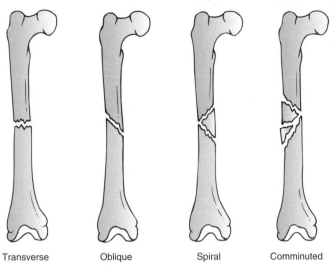

| Transverse | Oblique | Spiral | Comminuted |

Figure 1.6. Fracture patterns.

Greenstick

This fracture shape is seen in children, whose bones are covered by a thick periosteum layer, and are more elastic. An angulation force to this type of bone tends to bend the bone at one cortex and to buckle or break it at the other, thus producing an incomplete fracture. Although with severe violence young bones can suffer complete breaks, greenstick fractures are more commonly seen.

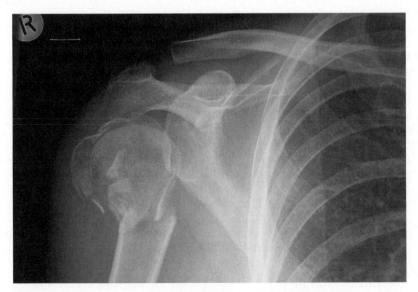

Figure 1.7. Comminuted fracture of the proximal humerus.

Intra-articular or extra-articular

Intra-articular

Fracture line extends into a joint surface

Extra-articular

Fracture line does not involve a joint surface.

Other commonly used terms include:

Impacted

The bone ends are pushed into each other.

Compression

This describes a bone that has been crushed and is most commonly used to refer to a collapsed vertebrae.

Thus a fracture may be classified by noting whether it is open or closed, displaced or undisplaced and by its shape, e.g. an open spiral displaced fracture of the mid-shaft of the right tibia. Fractures that are relatively common are sometimes known by a specific name, usually attributed to the surgeon who first described them. For instance, a Colles fracture is a specific fracture of the distal radius first described by Dr Abraham Colles.

Other more advanced forms of classification are used in the medical literature. These more complex systems are used to assist with surgical decision making and also in research. The Arbeitsgemeinschaft für Osteosynthesefragen (AO) system of fracture classification is commonly used by most surgeons and appears in the international literature. This allows for more accurate communication of fracture types between surgeons and comparison of different treatment methods.

Fracture healing

There are several described stages of fracture healing. The first stage is impact where energy is absorbed and failure occurs. This is followed by an induction stage where haematoma is formed at the fracture site, a fibrin clot is formed and there is release of chemical mediators. This results in an influx of inflammatory cells. Primary fracture callus (soft callus) that consists of cartilage and bone, is then formed below the periosteum. The conversion of this soft cartilaginous callus to woven bone by enchondral ossification is called hard callus formation and the exact process is influenced by the method of fracture treatment, the amount of movement at the fracture site and the gap between the fracture fragments. The woven bone is then remodelled over time to lamellar bone. There are four main ways that bone heals.

1. Primary fracture callus is seen with all methods of fixation and occurs 2 weeks following injury (periosteal soft callus). This is able

to bridge small gaps and is very tolerant of bone instability. Depending on the rigidity of the fracture fixation method used and any gaps between the fracture fragments, one of the following types of healing will occur.

2. External bridging callus occurs following cast immobilization and non-rigid intramedullary fixation. This is able to bridge fracture gaps and is very tolerant of movement. The cells migrate from the surrounding soft tissues and blood supply from periosteal vessels.
3. Late medullary callus requires bone stability and occurs with fixation using devices such as dynamic compression plates (DCP) and solid locked intramedullary nails with a stable fracture configuration. This is able to bridge the fracture gap if fixation is solid. This is slow healing and requires a blood supply from intramedullary vasculature.
4. Primary cortical healing only occurs if there is rigid fixation and no fracture gaps. This healing is slow, cannot bridge fracture gaps and needs an intact intramedullary blood supply. This represents primary remodelling with cutting cones and subsequent osteoid production.

Assessment of the progression of fracture healing is important in predicting when a bone is able to withstand normal loading. Several simple rules have been described to provide a rough estimate. Spiral fractures of the upper limb in children unites in 3 weeks, double for an adult, double for the lower limb, double for transverse fracture types and double for infection (Table 1.1). Therefore a transverse fracture of the tibia in an adult will unite in 24 weeks. Monitoring of the progression of fracture healing with clinical assessment and serial radiographs is important.

Table 1.1. Guidelines for time of fracture healing

Fracture type	Upper limb	Lower limb
Spiral unites	6 weeks	12 weeks
Spiral consolidates	12 weeks	24 weeks
Transverse unites	12 weeks	24 weeks
Transverse consolidates	24 weeks	48 weeks

Effect of metal fixation on fracture healing

In fractures that are internally fixated, the bone is dependent on the integrity of the implant due to the absence of external bridging callus. The implant diverts stress away from the fracture thus causing the bone to become locally osteoporotic and often it does not fully recover full strength until the implant is removed. Therefore with internal fixation, the healing process at the bone level is longer although the immediate strength of the fixation allows for early mobilization and return to normal function.

Factors affecting fracture healing

Age

In general the young heal faster than older people. With increasing age, bone becomes less stiff, less strong and more brittle with more porous material and fewer, thinner and longer trabeculae.

Fracture site

The upper limb heals faster than the lower limb.

Fracture shape

A transverse fracture takes longer to heal than a spiral fracture.

Blood supply to the fragments

The local blood supply to the bone may be interrupted, in some cases delaying fracture healing. This occurs most commonly around the head of femur, scaphoid and talus due to the precariousness of the blood supply.

Amount of displacement of the fractures

Fractures with greater displacement and comminution will take longer to heal than a simple undisplaced fracture.

Health and fitness

A balanced healthy diet is required for efficient fracture healing. Vitamin C is required for normal collagen matrix formation. Exercise increases fracture healing as long as the callus is not dislodged by extreme or excess activity. Long-term use of corticosteroids inhibits osteoblast differentiation therefore slowing the healing process. Infection, anaemia or hypoxia will slow fracture healing.

Type of bone

Healing time is usually quicker in trabecular bone because of the rich blood supply. Intra-articular fractures take longer to heal than extra-articular fractures due to the presence of synovial fluid hindering the formation of granular tissue.

Principles of fracture management

There are three fundamental orthopaedic principles in fracture management. These are reduction of the fracture, followed by immobilization of the fracture and preservation of function. How the surgeon achieves each of these principles is based on a number of interacting factors including patient presentation, fracture position and configuration, research, and mobility of the patient.

Reduction

The first principle of fracture management is for the orthopaedic surgeon to decide whether the fracture needs reducing. Reduction means attempting to restore the fragments of the fracture as close to the original shape and position as possible. If the fracture is not displaced, minimally displaced or the displacement is immaterial to the eventual outcome, the surgeon may decide not to perform a reduction.

Closed reduction

Closed reduction (CR) is performed by manipulation of the fragments without the need for a surgical incision. It usually is conducted under radiological control after the patient has undergone either a general or local anaesthetic.

Open reduction

When closed reduction has failed, or as a method of choice, the fracture is reduced under direct vision at an open operation. When open reduction (OR) is performed the fragments are usually then fixed internally (with pins or plates) to ensure that the fracture position is maintained. This procedure is performed for unstable fractures, multiple fractures and pathological fractures.

Immobilization

There are five basic methods for immobilizing a fracture to allow healing to take place. These are cast immobilization, internal fixation, external fixation, traction and splinting.

Casts

Casts are the standard method of immobilizing a fracture particularly after closed reduction. However, casts may also be used as an extra method to maintain fracture stability in cases that have been internally fixed. Traditionally casts are made of plaster of Paris (POP), however in the last few years, synthetic material is being used more regularly. Synthetic material, such as fibreglass, has the advantage of being lighter in weight and more durable but is more expensive than POP, which limits its widespread application.

If the patient is allowed to toe-touch weight-bear then a cast boot or walking heel may be worn to minimize damage to the cast. A walking heel is attached to the cast whereas a cast boot is applied on to the cast and can be removed (Fig. 1.8). Cast boots are generally better as they do

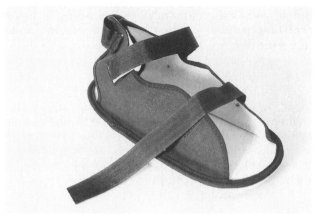

Figure 1.8. Cast boot.

not add height to the cast, allow a more normal gait pattern and protect the cast from external moisture and damage.

An important role of the physiotherapist following application of a cast is to assess the integrity of the circulation. When a cast has been applied over a fresh fracture or after an operation, circulation to the tissues above and below must be carefully monitored. Swelling within a closely fitting cast or splint may be sufficient to impede the venous return of the limb. The time of greatest danger is usually in the first 12–36 hours after injury.

Assessment should include:

- Pain in the limb out of proportion to that normally expected and not relieved with moderate analgesia.
- Inability to fully extend the fingers or toes.
- Assessment of distal sensation.
- Presence and strength of distal pulses (although the cast may prevent access).
- Assess warmth of distal extremity. Coolness of the distal extremity may indicate decreased circulation to the area.
- Blanching test. This assesses capillary refill by pressing on the nailbed for several seconds. If the blood supply is adequate then the nailbed should refill and become pink within several seconds of releasing the pressure.

Patients must be given instructions on how to care for their cast once they are discharged. The following instructions on an information sheet should be given:

- Pain in the limb should only be mild to moderate after cast application. If pain is severe and not relieved with oral analgesia, contact your doctor or physiotherapist immediately.
- Excessive swelling in the affected limb may cause the cast to feel tight. In the first few days following discharge from hospital the limb should be kept elevated.

- Move the fingers or toes regularly to prevent stiffness and maintain the effects of the muscle pump.
- Keep the cast dry. Cover the cast with a waterproof cover, such as a plastic bag, when showering or bathing.
- Do not insert objects, such as knitting needles, in to the cast in an attempt to relieve itching. This may cause scratches that may not heal.
- Regularly inspect the skin around the cast. If the skin below the cast changes colour, becomes numb, develops constant pins and needles or if the skin becomes very itchy, red and raw, contact your doctor or physiotherapist immediately.
- If the cast becomes soft, cracked or very loose, contact your doctor or physiotherapist immediately.

Traction

In some fractures, casts may be insufficient to hold the fracture, particularly those of the shaft of femur and tibia or lower humerus. Oblique and spiral fractures, due to the pull of strong large muscles drawing the fragments over one another, are not suited to cast immobilization. In such a case the action of the muscles can be balanced by traction on the distal limb. Traction is achieved by a mechanical pull, applied to either the skin (skin traction) or directly to the bone (skeletal traction). Skin traction is used when short periods of traction are required. Skeletal traction is used for longer periods. With skeletal traction, traction is applied through pins or tongs which are secured to the underlying bone. Traction is not common management choice as the methods for internal fixation are much improved.

The most commonly used traction devices are Hamilton–Russell traction, gallows traction and pelvic traction. Hamilton–Russell traction is used for fractures around the acetabulum and pelvis. Thus traction may be used in a patient following severe multiple trauma with associated lower limb fractures (Fig. 1.9). In young children, gallows traction is used to immobilize femoral shaft fractures, whilst in cases of multiple trauma that involves fractures of the pelvic ring, pelvic traction may be used (Fig. 1.10).

Internal fixation

Internal fixation (IF) is the most common method of holding a fracture. Internal fixation is generally used as a method of choice in certain fractures to secure immobilization and to allow early mobility. It is also used when it is impossible to maintain reduction by POP or traction alone and when it has been necessary to perform an open reduction.

Management with open reduction and internal fixation (ORIF) is the preferred treatment option as it decreases the length of stay in hospital, permits joint motion and early patient mobility. As a result there appears to be less risk of complications such as delayed and non-union.

The choice of methods will depend upon the site and pattern of fracture. Common types of internal fixation techniques are listed overleaf.

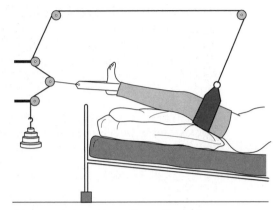

Figure 1.9. Hamilton–Russell traction.

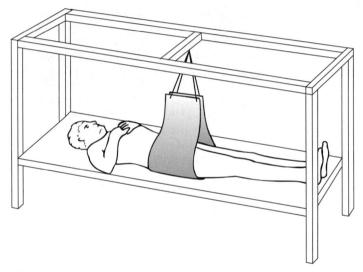

Figure 1.10. Pelvic traction.

Plate held by screws
Used for long bones, 4, 6 or 8 hole plates plus occasionally double plates.

Bone graft held by screws
A bone graft from another part of the body or stored bone from a bone bank is secured in place with screws. This is used for fractures with delayed or non-union.

Intramedullary nail
Intramedullary nails (IM) are used to hold fractures of the long bones, e.g. fractured shaft of tibia (Fig. 1.11).

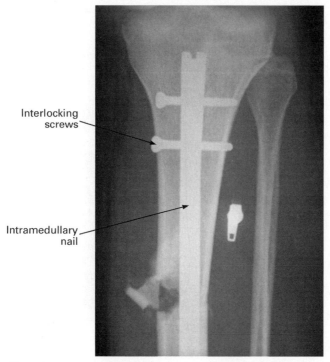

Interlocking
screws

Intramedullary
nail

Figure 1.11. Intramedullary nail for a fractured tibia.

Compression screw plate
Compression screw plates are a standard method of fixation for fractures of the neck of femur (Fig. 1.12). They are also known as dynamic hip screws (DHS). The screw component which grips the femoral head slides telescopically in the barrel, allowing the bone fragments to be held firmly together across the fracture.

Transfixion screws
Transfixion screws are used for the fixing of small fragments such as medial malleolus of tibia. A single screw usually suffices. They are usually placed at an angle and may be used for oblique or spiral fractures of long bones.

Circumferential wire bands
Originally this was a common method of internal fixation for oblique or spiral fractures. However, the wire bands were thought to strangle blood vessels in the periosteum, hindering or delaying union. Therefore they are not used commonly. Fractures of the patella are perhaps the only area where wire bands are used.

Metals used for internal fixation must be resistant to corrosion whilst in tissues. They are usually made of a special stainless steel (chromium and nickel alloy).

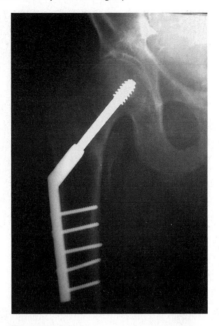

Figure 1.12. Compression screw
plate for fractured neck of femur.

External fixation

External fixation (EF) is a rigid support of bone fragments to an external
device, such as a metal bar, through the medium of pins inserted into the
fragments (Fig. 1.13).

EF is mainly used in open or infected fractures as it generally requires a
small incision. The use of IF devices, such as nails or plates, in these cases
carries a greater risk of promoting or exacerbating infection. External fixation also allows early movement of the joints above and below the fracture.

Splinting

Splinting is mainly used for undisplaced fractures of the metacarpals and
phalanges, e.g. buddy splinting two fingers together. Various types of
splints are also used following soft tissue reconstruction. There are a
variety of commercially made splints, such as the Zimmer splint that
can be applied post-operatively (Fig. 1.14).

Complications of fracture and soft tissue injury

Like classification of bone injury, the complications of fractures and soft
tissue injuries can be classified in different ways. They can be classified or
named by the time frame within which they occur or by the area affected.

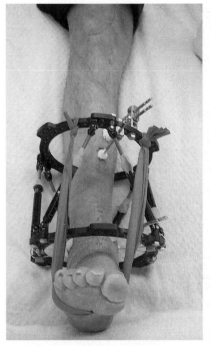

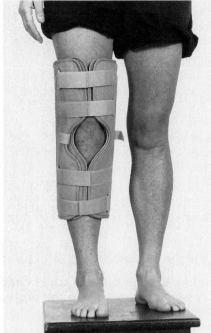

Figure 1.13. External fixation.   **Figure 1.14.** Zimmer splint.

Time frame

Immediate	Within a few hours
Early	Within the first few weeks
Late	Months and years later

Area

Local	In the region of the fracture or surgery
General	More systemic to injury and surgery

Only the immediate and early complications will be discussed as the aim of this book is to outline acute care management of patients following orthopaedic surgery.

Haemorrhage

Bones are vascular structures and therefore will haemorrhage or bleed when fractured. Apart from the blood lost from the bone itself, the sharp fracture ends may protrude into the surrounding soft tissue resulting in more blood loss. This resultant loss of blood affects the blood flow and tissue perfusion. As there is insufficient blood volume there will be a reduction in venous return with incomplete filling of the ventricular chambers of the heart. This will lead to insufficient cardiac output with a resultant fall in blood pressure and decreased tissue perfusion which leads to hypoxia, acidosis and progressive cell damage. Patients are then said to be in hypovolaemic shock.

Clinical features of hypovolaemic shock include:

- Breathing becomes rapid and shallow.
- Lips and skin become pale.
- Increased pulse rate.
- Drop in blood pressure.
- Patient becomes apathetic and thirsty.
- Eventually there is impaired renal function and urinary output decreased.

Treatment of hypovolaemic shock should include increasing the intra-vascular volume. Treatment should include control of further haemor-rhage and fluid replacement by parenteral fluids.

Damage to surrounding structures

Serious damage can also arise from damage to neighbouring soft tissues. For example, fractures to the ribs may cause perforation of a lung and result in a pneumothorax, whilst fractures of the vertebrae may cause damage to the spinal cord.

Damage to arterial blood vessels in the immediate vicinity may occur. The most common blood vessels to be affected are the brachial artery in supracondylar fractures of the humerus in children, the popliteal artery in fractures and dislocations at the knee and the aorta in fractures of the fourth and fifth thoracic vertebrae.

Nerves may also be affected. Common nerve injuries include the radial nerve in fractures of the humeral shaft and the peroneal nerve in fractures of the proximal fibula.

Nerve damage usually consists of a neuropraxia (physiological inter-ruption of the nerve) and is caused by direct compression or traction on the nerve or may be secondary to compression from splints. Recovery from a neuropraxia is almost always complete and takes several days to several weeks. Axonotmesis (incomplete division of the nerve) is usually secondary to traction on the limb and recovery may take several months depending on the distance from the injury to the distal nerve ending (30 day lag time and then 1 mm healing per day). Neurotmesis (complete division of the nerve) is rare after closed fractures but may occur with penetrating injuries or open fractures and nerve recovery is variable and often delayed. In closed fractures recovery is usual and should be awaited.

Wound infection

Wound infection following trauma is mainly limited to open fractures whereby the wound is contaminated by organisms carried into the body from an external source. In rare circumstances, a closed fracture may become infected inadvertently during the surgical procedure. The risk of infection is proportional to the severity of the fracture, extent of soft tissue damage, degree of wound contamination and time from injury to surgical debridement and antibiotics. There is a small risk that wound infection will extend to the underlying bone, giving rise to osteomyelitis. Bone infections will require adequate drainage, open debridement and antibiotic medication.

Infection after joint replacement surgery is a major concern; however, the incidence is less than 1 per cent. Risk factors include diabetes, obesity, rheumatoid arthritis, multiple previous surgeries and pre-existing urine or chest infection. A reduction in infection has been achieved with the combined use of clean air in operating theatres and systemic antibiotics. Infection following joint replacement is treated aggressively with surgical debridement and antibiotics.

Fracture blisters

These common blisters are seen after severe trauma with significant soft tissue damage and swelling. Severe soft tissue oedema causes an elevation of the superficial layers of skin. The blisters can sometimes be prevented by firm bandaging and should be treated by application of a dry dressing. To reduce the incidence of infection the blisters should not be broken.

Pressure sores

Prolonged bed rest or immobility of a limb due to pain or weakness may predispose to pressure sores. These are preventable by regular pressure area care with regular turns, good quality bedding and padding, care taken with transfers and regular inspection of potential pressure problem areas.

Fat embolism syndrome

The pathogenesis of fat embolism is controversial and still remains a poorly understood complication of skeletal trauma. The incidence in single long bone fractures is between 0.5 and 3.5 per cent and in multi-trauma is between 5 and 10 per cent. There are two main inter-related theories. A mechanical theory has been proposed where bone marrow and fat fragments are released into the peripheral circulation due to repeated manipulation or failure to splint the fracture. The fat droplets are deposited in the lungs causing a mechanical obstruction in the micro-circulation. More recent evidence suggests there is more to fat embolism than simple mechanical obstruction and a metabolic theory where fat embolism can occur by way of changes in the blood lipid profile has been suggested. This explains how the fat gets past the lungs from the venous system and results in systemic emboli. Fat in the microcirculation of the lungs causes release of lipase and the free fatty acids and glycerol that are toxic to the lung parenchyma and cause severe inflammation. This results in the release of chemotoxins and other mediators that cause tissue destruction in the lungs and other organs.

The clinical features of fat embolism syndrome include shortness of breath, restlessness and confusion. Fever and tachycardia are normally present whilst blood pressure is usually within normal limits in the acute stage. There is an associated anaemia, thrombocytopenia and elevated ESR and fat may be found in the venous blood or urine. A petechial rash on the front and back of the chest and neck and conjunctiva become evident on the second or third day after injury. Hypoxia is the hallmark of the fat embolism syndrome and may result in coma potentiated by cerebral emboli leading to cerebral oedema. Chest X-ray will show a progressively snowstorm like appearance with pulmonary infiltrations.

Preventative measures include adequate hydration, oxygenation and immobilization of fractured long bones in the immediate period. Treatment is directed towards oxygenation, haemodynamic support and early fixation of long bone fractures. Treatment in intensive care with ventilatory assistance may be required in order to maintain an adequate arterial oxygen tension. Use of massive intravenous steroid therapy and heparin have been advocated.

Chest infection

Chest infection can occur particularly in the elderly from being immobile. This is covered in more detail in Chapter 3.

Deep vein thrombosis and pulmonary embolus

Deep vein thrombosis and pulmonary embolism are serious, potentially life-threatening complications following orthopaedic surgery. This is covered in Chapter 3.

Compartment syndrome

The muscles of the upper and lower limbs consist of separate muscle groups that are each surrounded by a fascial (fibrous tissue) envelope attached to bone. Trauma to a bone or muscle may cause bleeding into each separate compartment of muscles that have a finite volume. Any further bleeding and swelling will result in increased pressure within the compartment that compromises the circulation and the function of the contents of that space (Fig. 1.15). Nerves will function for between 2–4 hours without a blood supply and peripheral nerves have the potential to recover. Muscle can last 6–8 hours without a blood supply but has no potential for regeneration once ischaemic and will heal with a fibrous scar.

Compartment syndrome should not be mistaken for transient pain, swelling and neurological loss caused by tight dressings or a plaster cast that is reversed by removal of the dressing or cast.

The first and most important symptom of an impending acute compartment syndrome is that pain is greater than expected from the primary problem, such as a fracture or contusion. The patient has a swollen, palpably tense limb and there is pain on passive stretching of the involved muscles. Paresis or weakness is an unreliable sign and may be secondary

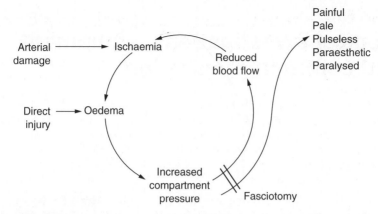

Figure 1.15. Cycle leading to development of compartment syndrome.

to nerve involvement, primary ischaemia, or guarding secondary to pain. Paraesthesia does not indicate the severity of the swelling and is nearly always present as each compartment of the arm or leg has at least one nerve passing through it. Unless major arterial injury or disease is present, in the early stages compartment syndrome, peripheral pulses are generally palpable and capillary refill is routinely present. However, as the pressure increases, capillary refill will be reduced resulting in skin pallor and peripheral pulses may be absent.

Treatment is by surgical release of the compartment fascia based on clinical suspicion and may be confirmed with direct measurement of the compartment pressure. The normal resting pressure of the limb tissue compartments is approximately 5 mmHg. Compartment syndrome occurs when tissue pressure increases to greater than 30–40 mmHg. The wounds are left open following release and will require further surgery to treat the muscle damage and obtain wound closure when the swelling has reduced. Skin grafting may be required to achieve wound closure.

CHAPTER 2

Medical investigations, equipment and common medication

This chapter outlines routine medical investigations and tests, patient attachments and selected medications. It is important that the physiotherapist has an understanding of specialized patient attachments and investigations in order to take the necessary precautions when treating patients. For similar reasons, physiotherapists should also have an awareness of the effects and adverse reactions of many of the common medications used following orthopaedic surgery.

Medical investigations

Vital signs

Blood pressure, pulse rate, respiration rate and body temperature are the most usual vital signs to be examined after orthopaedic surgery. Vital signs are usually measured routinely by nursing staff following orthopaedic surgery. The physiotherapists should check these prior to assessment and treatment of patients. Table 2.1 lists the accepted normal values for the vital signs. However there are variations from these norms amongst the population; thus it is important to check the pre-operative values to establish a norm for each patient.

Blood tests

There is an extensive list of blood tests that can be used to diagnose disease, complications and monitor a patient's response to treatment. There is an increasing requirement for doctors and other health professionals to be accountable for the rational use of investigations in hospital to reduce costs and improve patient management. Physiotherapists need to have an awareness of the results of blood tests that may impact on patients' exercise tolerance and compliance.

Complete blood examination (CBE)

A complete blood examination is usually performed as part of routine screening when a patient is admitted to hospital. This usually includes red and white cell counts, haemoglobin (Hb), erythrocyte indices and exam-

Table 2.1. Normal values of vital signs in adults

Vital sign	Normal value	Implication of abnormal values
Blood pressure	90/60–120/80 mmHg	If high, hypertensive patient may be stressed and anxious or already have high blood pressure. If low, patient may be hypotensive and require careful handling during any attempts to transfer or mobilize.
Pulse rate	50–100 beats/min	If higher than normal, could indicate patient stress and anxiety. Check for other co-morbid conditions and factors that could affect these, e.g. fluid depletion.
Respiration rate	12 breaths/min	
Body temperature	36–37.5°C	If high, then may indicate infection (wound, respiratory or urinary). However, temperature is often elevated for several days after surgery.

Table 2.2. Normal values and significance of abnormal values of relevant blood test factors

	Normal values	Physiotherapy significance of abnormal values
White blood cell count	$4–11 \times 10^9/l$	Increased range may indicate an infection of bacterial origin.
Haemoglobin (Hb)	Males: 13–18 g/100 ml. Females: 12–16 g/100 ml	A reduction in haemoglobin levels indicates anaemia or severe haemorrhage. Patients will fatigue easily.
Platelets	$150–450 \times 10^9/l$	Bruising may occur when the platelet count falls below $100 \times 10^9/l$. Severe bleeding tends to occur when the platelet count falls below $50 \times 10^9/l$.

ination of the peripheral blood cells. Table 2.2 outlines some normal values that are relevant to physiotherapists. Nursing staff take the blood sample from the hand or arm.

Post-operative anaemia is a common outcome of major orthopaedic operations. Treatment should be based on the Hb level, general health of the patient and current symptoms such as lethargy, dizziness and drowsiness. A Hb level less than 9 g/dl may be symptomatic and require transfusion although Hb levels down to 6 g/dl may be tolerated by some patients.

Most patients undergoing major elective surgery, such as total hip replacement, require post-operative transfusions to reduce the risk of post-operative anaemia. This is most commonly performed with autologous blood (patient's own, pre-donated blood). The use of autologous blood after elective surgery avoids the need for homologous blood (type-specific donor blood) that has a 10 per cent risk of adverse events. For instance, there is a 0.5 per cent risk per unit of homologous blood for transfusion transmitted diseases (HIV is transmitted in 1:1 000 000, Hepatitis B in 1:200 000 and Hepatitis C in 1:5000). Ninety per cent of autologous blood donors do not require homologous blood. For example, with total knee replacement (TKR), the likelihood of requiring homologous blood has decreased from 56 per cent to 5 per cent with autologous donation. However, it is four times the cost to donate autologous blood and 40–70 per cent of autologous units are not used.

General biochemistry

Most laboratories will perform a complete analysis of the common electrolytes, renal and hepatic function and bone minerals. This may be requested under the names MBA (multiple biochemical analysis) or LFT (liver function test). The normal values will vary between laboratories and are normally printed on the results page next to the measured values. Many results pages will have a few summary lines at the bottom of the page. Interpretation of biochemical abnormalities is beyond the scope of this book; however, drowsiness, confusion or irritability may be due to specific abnormalities and require medical review.

Attachments and equipment

Intravenous therapy (IVT)

Most patients will require intravenous fluids during the peri-operative period. Patients with medical problems such as renal impairment, cardiac failure, blood loss following trauma or surgery or dehydration require careful fluid management to ensure a normal circulating blood volume.

It is an advantage to adequately rehydrate patients prior to emergency surgery and in some cases (e.g. fractured NOF) surgery may be delayed until the patient is rehydrated or has received a blood transfusion. In some circumstances (e.g. pelvic fractures, major abdominal and chest trauma and open wounds) surgical intervention may be required to control blood loss and therefore takes priority.

The general rules for fluid replacement are to replace prior fluid loss (haemorrhage, dehydration, vomiting), allow for ongoing fluid loss (wound drainage, vomiting, fever) and provide normal maintenance of fluids (urine, general metabolism). It is therefore important to have accurate documentation of fluid input and output. It is also important to consider the electrolyte balance (mainly sodium, potassium, chloride and bicarbonate) of the body and have an understanding of the daily requirements and the amount of electrolytes in different fluids that have been lost and need replacement. By calculating both the fluid and electrolyte requirements, a fluid replacement plan can be developed. This requires regular close monitoring and adjustment. Although most orthopaedic patients do not have complex fluid losses, the elderly patient with a fractured neck of femur often has complex medical conditions that make fluid balance difficult.

Supplemental oxygen

Many patients require supplemental oxygen following trauma or surgery to improve tissue oxygenation to the brain, heart and traumatized tissues. Many patients have impaired diffusion of oxygen due to anaesthetic and analgesic medications, pulmonary atelectasis or infection, fat embolism and pulmonary embolism.

Patients with severe respiratory disease may retain carbon dioxide if given high levels of oxygen and therefore the percentage of inspired oxygen needs to be carefully controlled in these patients.

Oxygen saturation can be easily measured in the majority of patients with a transcutaneous fingertip monitor; however, accurate assessment of arterial oxygenation requires evaluation of an arterial blood sample in complex cases.

Urinary catheters

A urinary catheter may be used to remove urine from the bladder when the patient is unable to control the release or retention of urine. Urinary retention can be a complication following orthopaedic surgery particularly if epidural anaesthesia has been used. This is thought to be due to delayed recovery of the normal autonomic bladder reflexes.

Catheters can be applied externally or internally (also known as an indwelling catheter). An external catheter is only appropriate for males whereby a condom is applied over the penis and attached to an external drainage tube and bag. Internal catheters can be of two types: urethral catheter or suprapubic catheter. A urethral catheter is inserted via the urethra, past the internal sphincter into the bladder. A suprapubic catheter is inserted directly into the bladder via a small abdominal wall incision. Once in place the catheter may be sutured or held in place with tape. The presence of catheters should not interfere with physiotherapy treatment. The catheter drains due to the effect of gravity and thus should not be placed higher than the bladder for a long period.

In addition the catheter should be positioned carefully during any exercises and mobilization to reduce the risk of stretching, disconnection or discomfort.

Patient-controlled analgesia (PCA)

Any form of pain relief can be administered to the patient by patient-controlled analgesia. This method allows the patient to administer their own pain medication (commonly morphine) on demand and within the limits of safety. Most commonly this is performed through an intravenous unit. The system consists of a reservoir of medication connected to an intravenous (IV) line and is controlled by a small pump which the patient wears on the wrist. When the patient presses a button on the pump, a predetermined dose of medication is delivered. The pump is calibrated to only supply medication with specific time intervals to eliminate the risk of the patient overdosing. The pump can also record the amount of medication and the number of times that the patient has received the medication. If a patient is due to have physiotherapy treatment then they should be advised to press the button at least 20 minutes before treatment to gain maximum pain relief. The presence of PCA should not interfere with the patients' physiotherapy treatment. However care should be taken with the IV attachment during all mobilization and transfer activities.

Medication

This section has been included for general information only. Physiotherapists should be cognizant of the common medications used in musculoskeletal conditions and following orthopaedic surgery. Knowledge of the effect and potential adverse reactions is important when assessing or planning physiotherapy intervention. Although there are many reported interactions and adverse reactions for all medications, only the most common have been listed in this chapter. This section should not be used as a reference for prescribing medications.

Analgesics

Analgesia with narcotic analgesia, such as morphine and pethidine, is produced through an interaction between the narcotic analgesia and the narcotic receptors in the central nervous system. Analgesia occurs through an elevation of the patient's pain threshold and an alteration in the physical reaction to the painful stimuli. They are commonly used in the management of post-operative pain and may be given by small intravenous injections or intravenously. When pain is controlled, analgesia will be changed to oral analgesia, such as Panadeine Forte or Digesic.

Morphine and pethidine

Indications:	Moderate to severe pain.
Precautions:	Severe CNS depression.
	Poor respiratory function.
	May lead to dependence and tolerance.
	Pethidine is more addictive and may lead to problems of toxicity.
Adverse reactions:	Respiratory depression.
	Constipation, light headedness, sedation, nausea, vomiting, rash.

Physiotherapy implications
Narcotic analgesia suppresses normal respiration and therefore it is very important to perform deep breathing exercises and change position regularly to reduce the risk of respiratory post-operative complications. Narcotics can also cause some postural hypotension, therefore patients should be sat up slowly.

Panadeine Forte (paracetamol 500 mg, codeine 30 mg)

Indications:	Relief of moderate to severe pain.
Precautions:	Patients with hepatic or renal failure.
	Central nervous system (CNS) depression or poor respiratory function.
	Patients should not drive, operate machinery or drink alcohol whilst taking this medication.
Adverse reactions:	Nausea, vomiting, constipation and drowsiness.

Physiotherapy implications
Patients may experience the side effects of nausea, dizziness and drowsiness. This should be adequately assessed before ambulating or exercising a patient.

Digesic or Capadex (dextropropoxyphene 32.5 mg, paracetamol 325 mg)

Indications:	Relief of mild to moderate pain.
Precautions:	Patients with anaemia, hepatic or renal failure.
	Alcohol and other CNS depressants.
Adverse reactions:	Nausea, vomiting, sedation and dizziness.
	Weakness, euphoria and headache.

Physiotherapy implications
Patients may experience the side effects of nausea, dizziness and drowsiness. This should be adequately assessed before ambulating or exercising a patient.

Non-steroidal anti-inflammatory drugs (Feldene, Orudis, Naprosyn, Voltaren, Indocid, Celebrex)

Non-steroidal anti-inflammatory drugs (NSAIDs) are used for the relief of pain and inflammation in many different musculoskeletal conditions. Commonly they are used in the management of osteoarthritis, rheumatoid arthritis and sero-negative arthropathies such as ankylosing spondylitis.

Indications:	Symptomatic treatment of rheumatoid arthritis, osteoarthritis and ankylosing spondylitis.
Precautions:	Peptic ulceration, active gastro-intestinal bleeding or inflammation. There is a risk of gastro-intestinal bleeding and perforation in approximately 1–4 per cent of the population. Asthma and haemorrhagic tendencies.
Adverse reactions:	Gastro-intestinal side effects occur in 20 per cent of people. Dizziness and headache.

Physiotherapy implications
Patients may complain of gastro-intestinal pain or discomfort.

Anti-coagulant drugs

Following major orthopaedic surgery, it may be necessary to suppress the normal blood clotting mechanism of the body. Prophylactic anti-coagulant therapy may be administered to minimize the risk of developing a venous thromboembolism following surgery.

Clexane (Enoxaparin)

Indications:	Prevention of deep vein thrombosis (DVT) after major orthopaedic surgery. Treatment of established DVT.
Precautions:	Active peptic ulceration and ulcerative colitis, major bleeding disorders. Recent stroke.
Adverse reactions:	Haemorrhage. Thrombocytopaenia.

Warfarin

Indications:	DVT and pulmonary embolism (PE) prophylaxis and treatment.

Precautions:	Active peptic ulceration and ulcerative colitis, major bleeding disorders.
	Recent stroke.
	Dosage is unpredictable and requires careful monitoring to ensure a safe therapeutic range.
Adverse reactions:	Haemorrhage.
	Overdosage.

Aspirin (acetylsalicylic acid)

Indications:	DVT prophylaxis (aspirin has anti-coagulant properties when used in higher doses).
	Analgesia.
	Inflammation.
Precautions:	Alcohol.
	Peptic ulceration and bleeding tendencies.
	Asthma.
Adverse reactions:	Minor gastro-intestinal bleeding.

Physiotherapy implications

With all anti-coagulant medication, there is a slightly increased risk of bleeding. Physiotherapists should take extra care when handling patients during transfer and mobilization techniques. Any large haematoma development should be reported to the medical staff as there is a risk that the patient may be over anti-coagulated.

Anti-emetics

Anti-emetics are used for the control of nausea and vomiting. They do not treat the cause of nausea and vomiting but alleviate the symptoms. They may be used post-operatively if patients have a reaction to the general anaesthetic.

Maxolon (metoclopramide)

Indications:	Nausea and vomiting.
Precautions:	Dystonic reactions can occur (1 per cent).
Adverse reactions:	Drowsiness and fatigue.
	Headache and dizziness.

Physiotherapy implications

Patients may feel drowsy and fatigue easily.

Antibiotics

Antibiotics are substances produced by microorganisms that, in high dilution, are antagonistic to the growth of other microorganisms. Some antibiotics are made synthetically.

Cephalothin (1st generation cephalosporin)

Indications:	Treatment and prophylaxis of infection caused by *Staphylococci, Streptococci, Haemophilus* and *E. coli.*
Precautions:	Cross-allergy in patients with a penicillin allergy (5–10%).

Gentamicin

Indications:	Treatment and prophylaxis of gram negative infection.
Precautions:	Care with dosage in renal impairment because of nephrotoxicity and ototoxicity.
Adverse reactions:	Nephrotoxicity (renal toxicity). Ototoxicity (hearing loss).

Gastro-intestinal protective agents

Gastro-intestinal protective agents, such as Zantac, are commonly administered for the prevention and treatment of peptic ulceration and reflux oesophagitis. They are commonly prescribed in conjunction with NSAIDs to reduce the incidence of gastro-intestinal side effects seen with these drugs.

Zantac (ranitidine)

Indications:	Short-term and maintenance treatment of proven peptic ulceration.
Precautions:	May mask symptoms of carcinoma of the stomach. Adverse reactions: Headache. Constipation and diarrhoea.

Physiotherapy implications
Although it is rare to have side effects, take care when mobilizing and exercising patients as diarrhoea, tiredness and lethargy can be experienced.

CHAPTER 3

Principles of physiotherapy assessment and management

The physiotherapist on an orthopaedic ward will treat patients who have been admitted for a variety of different reasons. Patients can be admitted as an elective admission, that is, a planned operation such as a total knee replacement, or an acute admission, for example, following a traumatic incident that requires surgery or other forms of medical intervention. This chapter aims to describe principles of physiotherapy assessment and management that are common to all patients.

Physiotherapy assessment

For each patient, the physiotherapist will need to perform a detailed assessment in order to define the patient's problems accurately. Assessment is based on the subjective and objective information gained from the patient and additional information from the medical records. The physiotherapy assessment should follow the SOAP format. This should include the following information:

S   Subjective assessment
     Subjective information will include information gained from interviewing the patient or relatives. Information that should be gained should include: previous mobility levels, social support, steps and stairs at home, current pain levels, cardiorespiratory status, general health, comorbid conditions.

O   Objective assessment
     Objective assessment will measure the physical status of the patient. Physiotherapists will need to evaluate muscle strength, range of movement, general fitness and health, cardiovascular status.

A   Assessment
     A statement should be made on the patient's general health and recovery as well as the operative procedure. Any factors that may limit the patient's recovery should be noted.

P   Plan
     This should outline the expected progression of the rehabilitation, in particular, exercises and mobility progression.

Any plans or arrangements to be made for the patient's discharge should also be included.

This is usually followed by:

Rx   Treatment
An outline of the treatment performed including exercises, transfers and mobility.

Documentation

The assessment and all follow-up treatment needs to be accurately and concisely recorded in the patient's medical records. Most hospitals in Australia use the Problem-Oriented Medical Record (POMR). This system organizes the medical record using a common list of patient problems as its base (Weed, 1968). The POMR collates subjective and objective information as well as laboratory tests gained from the patient. This information is organized in the case notes into five sections. These sections are: Database, Problem List, Plans, Progress Notes and Discharge Summary (details provided in Table 3.1). All associated medical professions document their assessment and treatment in the patient's medical record pertaining to the patient's problem list. This will include documentation by the orthopaedic surgeon, nursing staff and all allied health professionals including physiotherapists, occupational therapists and social workers. The results of all investigations including blood tests, radiological investigations such as radiographs and computerized tomography (CT) scans are also maintained in the patient's medical records.

All documentation included in the medical record can become a legal document in a litigation proceeding, so they should therefore be an accurate reflection of the assessment and treatment. The information contained in the medical record should allow the physiotherapist to accurately reconstruct the treatment episode without the recourse to memory. As the risk of litigation is gradually increasing, the following principles when documenting assessment and treatment should be applied:

- All entries should be legible and easily understood so that another physiotherapist can assume management of the patient in the event of unexpected absence.
- Only standard and recognizable abbreviations should be used. A list of the most commonly used abbreviations can be found in the preliminary section.
- All entries should be dated and signed such that the physiotherapist's name is easily ascertained.
- Identify that the patient was informed of the treatment they were to receive and any particular risks associated with treatment. It is important to document that the patient understood this information and that they consented to treatment. Likewise it is important to document any refusal of treatment.
- Never leave spaces between lines in the case notes.
- Always use a blue or black pen.

Table 3.1. Details of sections of the POMR

Sections of POMR	Detail contained
Database	Contains core information about the patient. Includes patient demographics, history, physical data and laboratory tests and special investigations.
Problem list	A list of the patient's problems determined by the patient, clinician or both. Problems may be classified as medical, social, psychological, demographic or functional.
Initial plans	The plan is devised based on the problem list. The plan should include short- and long-term aims. Each plan should be directed at solving a particular problem. The plan may include further tests or investigations, or physiotherapy intervention.
Progress notes	These notes are written consecutively by all relevant members of the team including nursing, medical and physiotherapy staff. The notes should be written in the SOAP format with a summary of the patient's progress.
Discharge summary	When the patient is discharged from hospital, a discharge summary should be written in the case notes. If the patient is being transferred to another institution then a copy should be sent to that institution.

- Any alteration to an entry should be made by drawing a single line through the incorrect statement(s) followed by signing and dating of the correct information. If necessary ask another staff member to counter-sign the entry.
- Avoid the use of general and ambiguous statements. For example: 'Patient refused treatment' is too general and should be replaced by 'patient refused to be mobilized due to pain'.

Example of assessment and follow-up physiotherapy case note entry.
10.01.01
10.30 am
S: *Presenting complaint*
68-year-old lady admitted 09.01.01 for #NOF. Surgery last night – AMP. No surgical or post-operative complications to date. IDC and PCA in situ.
PCA working and present pain level about 4/10. No nausea or vomiting.
Patient understood and consented to physiotherapy treatment.

Past medical history
GH – good. High blood pressure.
(L) TKR for OA in 1996. No problems. Previous mobility – used a walking stick for long distances.
No previous cardiorespiratory problems.

Social history
Patient lives with her husband in ground floor flat – one small step in front door. No stairs. Daughter lives near by and good support.
Plays lawn bowls and active gardener – wants to get back.

O: F and A movts ✓ ✓ – no signs of DVT.
       C W M S ✓ ✓
       DB&C – good expansion.
       Cough – dry, non-productive, strong, effective.
       Quads – moderate static quads contraction.
       IRQ – unable to achieve due to pain and fatigue.
       Static gluteals – strong contraction.
       Active assisted hip flexion – 30° limited by pain.
A: 1 day post R AMP for # NOF – uncomplicated recovery.
       Pleasant, active and cooperative lady.
Rx: DB&C, F&A.
       Bed Exs – SQ, SG – exs sheet given to patient.
       Active assisted flexion.
       SOOB – transferred to chair × 2 MA. Felt a bit light headed.
       Stood and PWB few steps with frame.
Plan: Continue mobility – mobilize again this afternoon.
       Increase exercises – add assisted hip abduction and bridging.

11.01.01
S: Feeling brighter today. Has been showered. PCA and IDC removed. Pain 4/10.
       Eager to do exercises and to be mobile.
O: Active assisted hip flexion 40°.
       Quads contraction stronger. IRQ – 5° lag.
       Active assisted hip abduction 10°.
A: 1 day post AMP doing well.
P: Add bridging and teach step before goes home. ? D/C on Friday.
Rx: Walked 5 metres with frame WBAT.
       SOOB × 1 LA.
       Exercises.

Prophylactic physiotherapy techniques

Effective post-operative physiotherapy management requires a sound knowledge of the many surgical procedures, clear clinical reasoning and communication with all health providers as well as the patient. There are, however, post-operative physiotherapy techniques that are common to all patients who have undergone surgery or have been admitted for bed rest and observation. In these instances, elements of the physiotherapy post-operative management can be universally applied to all patients on an orthopaedic ward. The aim of management in these instances is to prevent the occurrence of post-operative complications that may delay or limit the patient's recovery.

Cardiorespiratory complications

Post-operative cardiorespiratory complications are a leading cause of post-operative morbidity and death, especially in the elderly (Iwamoto et al., 1993; Martin et al., 1984). Cardiorespiratory complications may follow any operation in which a general anaesthetic has been performed. The two main complications are atelectasis and bronchopneumonia.

Atelectasis is defined as closure or collapse of alveoli. It generally occurs post-operatively in the bases of the lungs. This may be seen on chest radiographs with a loss of normal lung volume. If not treated effectively atelectasis could lead to the development of pneumonia whereby infection of the lobes distal to the collapsed or closed alveoli occurs.

The risk of developing atelectasis and/or pneumonia following general anaesthetic is thought to be due to a number of factors:

1. Inhibition of the cough reflex. This may be due to the use of post-operative sedation or analgesia. In addition pain may inhibit the cough reflex particularly if the operative site is in close proximity to the abdomen or thorax.
2. Inhibition of normal muco-cilial clearance due to the general anaesthetic (GA) (Brooks-Bunn, 1995). This can result in a reduction in the elimination of normal respiratory secretions. Cilial action has been shown to cease for 90 minutes after a GA (Lunn, 1991).
3. Reduction in the functional residual capacity (FRC) which may be lowered by as much as 20 per cent for up to 24 hours after a GA (Sykes and Bowe, 1993). This is thought to last for several days after the surgery and to be related to diaphragmatic dysfunction due to reflex inhibition of phrenic nerve output (Ridley, 1998). Post-operative sedation can also result in upper chest breathing which, when combined with lengthy time-periods in a slumped position may limit effective excursion of the diaphragm.

Due to this limited ventilation, reduction in the action of the cilia and a depressed cough reflex, any respiratory secretions may not be cleared sufficiently. These secretions, when not effectively cleared, may form a mucous plug which has the potential to obstruct one of the airways resulting in further lung collapse. This can then lead to bronchopneumonia due to infection and inflammation of the mucous plug extending to the walls of the lungs. Common signs and symptoms of atelectasis include decreased breath sounds, crackles, cough, sputum production and, if left untreated, radiological evidence.

Patients who are identified to be at risk from the effects of a GA, e.g. those with existing respiratory dysfunction, may be selected to have a spinal anaesthetic, the most common example being an epidural placed between the third and fourth lumbar vertebrae.

The role of the physiotherapist is to assess the respiratory function of each patient pre-operatively in elective admissions or immediately post-operatively in cases of acute admissions. If the patient is admitted for an elective procedure this assessment should be performed at the pre-operative clinic. Patients admitted with trauma should be assessed as soon as possible following surgery. Questions regarding the patient's general health, smoking habits, respiratory history and medications should be included in the subjective examination. Other risk factors include: pre-existing chest infections, smoking history, reduced mobility, patient with rheumatological diseases affecting the costovertebral joints (e.g. ankylosing spondylitis), obesity, poor nutritional status and patients over 65 years (Ridley, 1998).

Following an operation all patients should be asked to perform full inspiration exercises, and must be asked to cough. This should be performed the day after the surgery. Coughing should only be performed with appropriate wound support and optimal pain management. Any patient with pre-existing cardiovascular disease requires careful assessment and ongoing monitoring. Patients who are generally healthy, young and have no pre-existing respiratory disease will require prophylactic chest physiotherapy. Breathing exercises should be performed on the first post-operative day but can be discontinued once the physiotherapist is satisfied that the chest is clear and that the patient is mobilizing well.

Deep breathe and cough exercises

- The patient should be positioned sitting upright, taking care of the surgical incision and operative site.
- The exercises should be explained and demonstrated to the patient first.
- The physiotherapist's hands should be placed either side of the chest wall usually one hand span below axilla. This provides proprioceptive input to stimulate movement of the chest wall (Fig. 3.1).
- The patient should be encouraged to relax their shoulders and there should be no scapular elevation when performing these exercises.
- The patient should be instructed to 'breathe in through your nose and push my hands away with your rib cage. Hold the breath for 2 seconds, then exhale through your mouth'.
- Ensure the patient is performing the technique correctly.
- Ask the patient to repeat this exercise three or four times, then rest.
- Take care not to hyperventilate the patient.
- Then instruct the patient to perform a deep, double cough from the bottom of the lungs. It is often useful to demonstrate this to the patient.
- If the cough is moist and productive, the cough should be repeated until clear (or as much as the patient can tolerate).
- Patients should repeat these breathing exercises two or three times every hour whilst on bed rest.

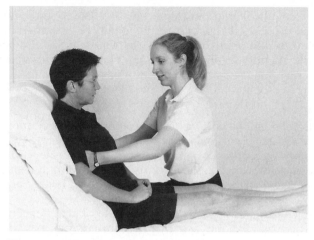

Figure 3.1. Position of hands for deep breathing exercise and instruction.

The physiotherapist should ascertain and record the nature of the cough. There are four main ways to describe the type of cough.

1. Effective or ineffective.
2. Moist or dry.
3. Strong or weak.
4. Productive or non-productive.

The type of cough and any sputum production should be recorded in the patient's case notes to alert medical staff to the possibility of cardio-respiratory complications. Patients who have retained secretions and who are unable to clear these effectively may need more specialized techniques. These techniques include active cycle of breathing techniques, shaking, percussion, and gravity-assisted positioning. A description of these techniques is beyond the scope of this book. The reader is referred to Webber and Pryor (1998).

Deep vein thrombosis and pulmonary embolism

There are three main factors that enhance thrombosis (blood clot) formation in the deep venous system of the lower limb. These include:

1. Venous stasis due to an immobile limb during prolonged bed rest or during the surgical procedure where the immobility or pressure on veins reduces the speed of blood flow. Warwick et al. (1994) demonstrated the cessation of blood flow in the femoral veins in 10 subjects with sustained flexion and adduction required during a total hip replacement procedure. Prolonged bed rest may also lead to decreased venous return due to poor diaphragmatic breathing and reduced chest expansion.

2. Hypercoagulability of the blood due to enhanced local and systemic activation of coagulation factors. Following an operation the number of platelets and their cohesiveness increases. It has also been found that the quantity of fibrinogen in the blood increases and there is a temporary suppression of the fibrinolytic system.
3. Damage to the intimal lining of the blood vessels due to the trauma of injury or positioning of the limb during surgery.

Venous thrombo-embolism is a serious potential complication of major orthopaedic trauma, joint replacement and spinal surgery. The incidence has been reported to be between 10 and 80 per cent depending on the method of detection and associated risk factors (Grady-Benson et al., 1994; Haake and Berkman, 1989; Haas et al., 1990; Salzman and Harris, 1976).

Deep veined thrombosis (DVT) may cause local symptoms of pain and swelling. There is also the risk that the thrombosis may detach and propagate to the lungs via the right side of the heart resulting in pulmonary embolism (PE) or, in the long term, may cause problems with post-phlebitic syndrome and venous insufficiency. The incidence of fatal PE is 0.1 per cent and the death rate following total hip replacement (THR) is 0.4 per cent (Salvati et al., 2000).

Important factors that increase the risk of development of venous thrombo-embolism include:

1. Prior DVT.
2. Prolonged immobilization.
3. Obesity.
4. Smoking.
5. Malignancy.
6. Oestrogen therapy.
7. Varicose veins.
8. Cardiac dysfunction.
9. Chronic respiratory disease.

Diagnosis of DVT

Diagnosis of DVT by clinical history and examination is difficult and is often inaccurate. Clinical features suggestive of DVT are an aching or cramp-like pain in the calf or behind the knee, tenderness on deep palpation, swelling of the lower limb and increased pain in the calf on passive dorsiflexion of the foot. This is known as Homan's sign (Fig. 3.2). However, many orthopaedic patients have swelling and discomfort in the lower limbs and movement of the ankle and knee may result in pain in the lower limb. DVT is currently diagnosed by having a high index of suspicion on clinical testing and by imaging with duplex ultrasound or venography of the lower limbs. Detection from a blood test is currently being evaluated.

Signs of pulmonary embolus development include:

- Hypoxia (low oxygen levels in the lung, blood and/or tissues).
- Tachypnoea (increased respiratory rate).

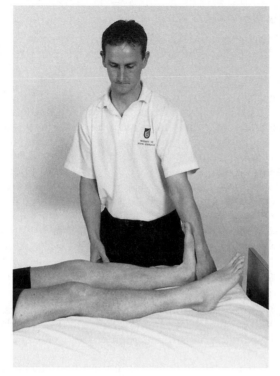

Figure 3.2. Homan's sign.

- Tachycardia (increased heart rate).
- Dyspnoea or shortness of breath (SOB).
- Sudden onset of severe chest wall pain, worse with deep inspiration or cough.

Prophylactic measures

Pharmacological prophylaxis is effective and most surgeons commence patients undergoing major elective surgery on pre-operative prophylactic medication, such as warfarin, clexane or aspirin to prevent the formation of DVT.

Other measures include the use of pneumatic compression devices during surgery and post-operative application of compression stockings. Research suggests that the use of pneumatic compression devices prevents the formation of DVT and may protect against pulmonary embolism, and reduce mortality (Haas et al., 1990; Salzman and Harris, 1976; Spain et al., 1998). It is important that mechanical devices or compression stockings be fitted correctly and function to increase the local venous return. Poorly fitted compression stockings have been shown to produce reverse pressure gradients and increase the incidence of DVT (Best et al., 2000).

Physiotherapy prophylaxis

Physiotherapy in the form of bed exercises and early mobilization helps to prevent DVT. The rationale behind bed exercises is that the venous circulation is assisted by action of the muscle pumps in the lower legs. Although there is no direct clinical evidence substantiating this hypothesis, research has shown that foot exercises alter blood flow in the lower legs. McNally et al. (1997) performed a randomized controlled trial to determine the effect of active foot movement 4 days after total hip replacement. Results demonstrated that venous outflow was increased after 1 minute of movement of the foot. In addition, Sochart and Hardinge (1999) found that active foot and ankle exercise produced higher peak and mean velocities of blood flow than passive exercise in a group of normal subjects. These studies confirm the beneficial haemodynamic effects of active movement of the foot in the post-operative period. Studies have also demonstrated that mobilization of THR patients on day one post-operatively reduces the incidence of DVT (Salvati et al., 2000).

Foot and ankle exercises (F&A)

- Explain the procedure to the patient.
- Ask them to bilaterally dorsiflex their feet. 'Pull your feet right up to point at your nose and then point them right down to the end of the bed.' Make sure the patient gets their ankles to the end of the active range each time.
- Then ask them to 'circle their feet around first clockwise then anti-clockwise'.
- If the patient has a lower leg cast in place, ask them to flex and extend their toes. Or if possible flex and extend their knee.
- Monitor and note any tenderness and warmth in the calf. Palpate along the calf (proximal to distal) for any signs of DVT (Fig. 3.3).
- Patients should repeat these exercises every hour whilst they are on bed rest.

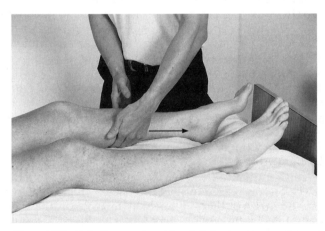

Figure 3.3. Palpate proximal to distal when assessing for a DVT.

Exercises
Generally, exercises for the unaffected leg/arm or other areas can and should be given to each patient for the length of their immobilization. This is of particular importance for patients who are on a long period of bed rest, e.g. traction. These exercises will help to prevent atrophy of the unaffected muscles and stiffness of unaffected joints. Of particular importance are the anti-gravity muscles required for standing and walking, e.g. inner range quads and gluteals. In addition regular re-positioning and turning will assist in the prevention of atelectasis as well as preventing the development of pressure areas.

For patients on long-term bed rest, muscle exercises to the unaffected limb(s) should be performed regularly. This will prevent muscle atrophy whilst also maintaining cardiovascular fitness. Pulleys and weights can be attached to a bed frame so that exercises can be performed.

Care maps or pathways

Healthcare budgets are becoming increasingly restricted and require all health care professionals to be more accountable and efficient for the services they provide and the patient outcomes that are produced. Hospital administrators are seeking to reduce the length of hospital stay in order to reduce the financial burden whilst at the same time attempting to improve patient outcomes. To achieve this, tools have been devised to outline and evaluate the provision of patient care. Such a tool is the patient care map (also known as care or critical pathways).

Care maps or critical pathways have been devised for a number of orthopaedic interventions including total hip and knee replacement. Care maps should be written in collaboration with all relevant health care workers including the orthopaedic surgeon, nurses, physiotherapist, occupational therapist and social worker. Development of the care map involves determining time-frames for key events, delineating standards for care and intervention during the entire hospital stay. This is then translated into a day-to-day framework or map so that patient goals can be identified and met each day. Apart from providing streamlined and standardized care, care maps also permit the recognition of factors that may interfere with the patient's progress and management initiated accordingly. An example of a care map is outlined in Table 3.2.

Care maps have been demonstrated to improve patient outcomes and decrease length of hospital stay after total knee and hip replacement (Dowsey et al., 1999; Gregor et al., 1996).

Patient education

Patient education is an essential component in the physiotherapy management of patients undergoing orthopaedic surgery. Pre-operative training and education in the operative procedure, exercise prescription and the use of assistive devices are an integral component of the rehabilitation process. Fear and anxiety can be allayed whilst a knowledge of what to

Table 3.2. Example of a care map for a total knee replacement

Care path	Day 1 (operating day)	Day 2 (Post-op day 1)	Day 3	Day 4	Day 5	Day 6
Consults		Surgeon, physiotherapy, case manager	Social work, physiotherapy	Surgeon, physiotherapy	Surgeon, physiotherapy	Surgeon, physiotherapy
Investigations	Post-operative XR	Hb taken, results checked	INR performed, results checked		INR performed, results checked	Complete blood picture checked
Medications	IV fluids, IV antibiotics, PCA analgesia, oxygen administered	IV fluids, IV antibiotics, PCA analgesia	Oral analgesia	Oral analgesia maintained	Oral analgesia maintained	Oral analgesia decreased
Wound drainage and dressing		Drain wound, dressing dry and intact	Drain removed, dressing dry and intact	Dressing dry and intact	Wound inspected	Wound inspected
Observations	Routine post-operative observations within normal limits	Routine post-operative observations within normal limits	Routine post-operative observations within normal limits	4/24 observations within normal limits	4/24 observations within normal limits	4/24 observations within normal limits

Activity	Bed rest, assist with deep breath and cough exercises, foot and ankle. CPM if ordered by doctor	Physiotherapy exercises, out of bed WBAT with frame. Continue DB&C, F&A and add other exercises	Walk 3 metres and continue exercises	Walk 5 metres and continue exercises	Walk independently and teach transfer techniques	Walk independently and teach steps and stairs
Education		Reinforce physiotherapy instructions	Reinforce physiotherapy instructions	Reinforce physiotherapy instructions	Educate on transfer techniques	Teach stairs
Discharge planning			Home needs discussed and organized. Convalescence bed booked if required	Discharge advice re ambulation, wound management, medication		Ready for discharge. Appointments made for follow-up with surgeon and physiotherapy

expect can have a profound effect on the patient's post-operative performance (Haines and Vieldion, 1990; Hathaway, 1986).

As the length of hospital stay for patients following most orthopaedic procedures is being reduced, physiotherapists have a limited time-frame in which to conduct patient education. For example, the length of stay for acute care following a hip fracture has decreased substantially in the 1980s and 1990s from 11 days to presently lasting between 3–5 days (Burns, 1996; Thomas, 1996). Because patients are being discharged earlier they must therefore have sufficient information to be responsible for their own post-operative care. Patient education in an acute care setting should not be much different than in other teaching settings. However, lack of time means that physiotherapists, along with other team members, must provide a more streamlined approach to patient education. Ruzicki (1989) outlined some simple yet effective ways to achieve this:

- A detailed patient assessment. This will help determine how much information the patient needs to know. For example, a patient who has had a left total hip replacement 6 months prior to having the right hip replaced, will know more about the recovery than a patient who is undergoing their first operation.
- 'Need to know' survival content. Provide simple essential information during the in-patient stay. A simple explanation of the surgery, using radiographs or operative photographs (which are now frequently available from arthroscopic techniques) or diagrams are important. Clear concise information about the exercises to perform until they are next reviewed should also be given.
- Instructions should be simple, concise and organized in a logical sequence.
- Printed media. Informational and instructional detail can be contained in pamphlets and brochures. This should include diagrams of exercises and activities that should be avoided.
- Involve family members, where possible, in the educative process.

Exercise prescription and discharge information

Patients should be discharged with sufficient information in both their post-operative exercises and information on any particular activities that must be avoided. In most hospitals, physiotherapists have standard post-operative hand-outs or booklets for the common surgical procedures. These should have been designed in collaboration with the operating surgeons and should be given to the patient prior to discharge. A contact phone number should be included with this information so that the patient has someone to contact if they are concerned about their progress.

Discharge information and exercise prescription on hand-outs needs to be presented to patients in a clear, understandable and motivating manner. Chapman and Langridge (1997) performed an analysis of 33 different hand-outs used by physiotherapists and found that 33 per cent of hand-outs were written well below the recommended reading level for health education literature. Chapman and Langridge (1997) suggest the following key points to consider when designing hand-outs or leaflets for patient education:

- Keep sentences and paragraphs short.
- Define technical and specialized words.
- Place emphasis on *key* points.
- Use illustrations where possible, and place them alongside relevant text.
- Use present tense, an active voice and a conversational style.

Patients may require on-going physiotherapy, therefore a detailed letter outlining all of the acute care management should be sent to the relevant physiotherapist. This will allow continuity of care.

References

Best, A. J., Williams, S., Crozier, A., Bhatt, R., et al. (2000). Graded compression stockings in elective orthopaedic surgery: An assessment of the in vivo performance of commercially available stockings in patients having hip and knee arthroplasty. *J. Bone Joint Surg.*, **82B**, 116–118.

Brooks-Bunn, J. A. (1995). Post-operative atelectasis and pneumonia. *Heart and Lung*, **24**, 94–115.

Burns, D. (1996). Appendix: collaborative pathway reports. *Topics in Geriatric Rehabilitation*, **12**, 77–89.

Chapman, J. A. and Langridge, J. (1997). Physiotherapy health education literature. *Physiotherapy*, **83**, 406–412.

Dowsey, M. M., Kilgour, M. L., Santamaria, N. M and Choong, P. F. M. (1999). Clinical pathways in hip and knee arthroplasty a prospective randomised controlled study. *Med. J. Austral.*, **170**, 59–62.

Grady-Benson, J. C., Oishi, C. S., Hanson, P. B., Colwell, C. W. et al. (1994). Post-operative surveillance for deep vein thrombosis with duplex ultrasonography after total knee arthroplasty. *J. Bone Joint Surg.*, **76A**, 1649–1657.

Gregor, C., Pope, S., Werry, D. and Dodek, P. (1996). Reduced length of stay and improved appropriateness of care with a clinical path for total knee or hip arthroplasty. *Joint Commiss. J. Qual. Improv.*, **22**, 617–628.

Haake, D. A. and Berkman, S. A. (1989). Venous thromboembolic disease after hip surgery. Risk factors, prophylaxis and diagnosis. *Clin. Orthop.*, **242**, 212–231.

Haas, S. B., Insall, J. N., Scuderi, G. R., Windsor, R. E. et al. (1990). Pneumatic sequential-compression boots compared with aspirin prophylaxis of deep-vein thrombosis after total knee arthroplasty. *J. Bone Joint Surg.*, **72A,** 27–31.

Haines, N. and Vieldion, G. (1990). A successful combination preadmission testing and pre-operative education. *Orthopaedic Nursing*, **9**. 53–57.

Hathaway, D. (1986). Effect of pre-operative instruction on post-operative outcomes – a meta-analysis. *Nursing Res.*, **35,** 269–275.

Iwamoto, K., Ichiyama, S., Shimokata, K. and Nakashima, N. (1993). Post-operative pneumonia in elderly patients: incidence and mortality in comparison with younger patients. *Int. Med.*, **32**, 274–277.

Lunn, J. N. (1991). *Lecture Notes on Anaesthesia*. Blackwell Science Publications.

Martin, L. F., Asher, E. F., Casy, J. M. and Fry, D. E. (1984). Post-operative pneumonia: determinants of mortality. *Arch. Surg.*, **119**, 379–383.

McNally, M. A., Cooke, E. A. and Mollan, R. A. (1997). The effect of active movement of the foot on venous blood flow after total hip replacement. *J. Bone Joint Surg.*, **79**, 1198–1201.

Ridley, S. C. (1998). Surgery for adults. In *Physiotherapy for Respiratory and Cardiac Problems* (J. A. Pryor and B. A. Webber, eds.) pp. 295–328, Churchill Livingstone.

Ruzicki, D. A. (1989). Realistically meeting the educational needs of hospitalised acute and short stay patients. *Nursing Clinics of North America*, **24**, 629–632.

Salvati, E. A., Pellegrini Jr., V. D., Sharrock, N. E., Lotke, P. A. et al. (2000). Symposium – recent advances in venous thromboembolic prophylaxis during and after total hip replacement. *J. Bone Joint Surg.*, **82A**, 252–270.

Salzman, E. W. and Harris, W. H. (1976). Prevention of venous thromboembolism in orthopaedic patients. *J. Bone Joint Surg.*, **58A**, 903–913.

Sochart, D. H. and Hardinge, K. (1999). The relationship of foot and ankle movements to venous return in the lower limb. *J. Bone Joint Surg.*, **81B**, 700–704.

Spain, D. A., Bergamini, T. M., Hoffman, J. F., Carillo, E. H. and Richardson, J. D. (1998). Comparison of sequential compression devices and foot pumps for prophylaxis of deep venous thrombosis in high risk trauma patients. *Amer. J. Surg.* **64**, 522–526.

Sykes, L. A. and Bowe, E. A. (1993). Cardiorespiratory effects of anaesthesia. *Clin. Chest Med.*, **14**, 211–216.

Thomas, R. L. (1996). Management of hip fracture in the geriatric patient – a team approach in the institutional setting. *Top. Geriat. Rehab.*, **12**, 59–69.

Warwick, D., Martin, A. G., Glew, D. and Bannister, G. C. (1994). Measurement of femoral vein blood flow during total hip replacement. Duplex ultrasound imaging with and without the use of a foot pump. *J. Bone Joint Surg.*, **76B**, 918–921.

Webber, B. A. and Pryor, J. A. (1998). Physiotherapy techniques. In *Physiotherapy for Respiratory and Cardiac Problems*. (J. A. Pryor and B. A. Webber, eds.) pp. 137–210, Churchill Livingstone.

Weed, L. L. (1968). Medical records that guide and teach. *New Engl. J. Med.*, **279**, 593–600, 652–657.

CHAPTER 4

Gait and mobility education

Trauma, disease or fatigue can all impact on a person's ability to mobilize and exercise. The physiotherapist working on an orthopaedic ward is responsible for the prescription, supply and instruction in the use of walking aids for the re-education of mobilization (Simpson and Pirrie, 1991). Physiotherapists are generally the first team member to assist the patient out of bed to a standing or sitting position. Following major surgery this can be a daunting task for both patient and therapist alike. This chapter describes the different mobilizing aids and techniques. Each technique can and should be adapted to suit different patients and surgical approaches.

Gait education

Definitions

NWB	Non-weight bearing
PWB	Partial weight bearing. This can vary from only a few kilograms to nearly all of the weight taken through the affected leg. Some surgeons are very specific regarding the amount of weight to be borne, e.g. no more than 20 kg. In these instances, a set of bathroom scales will be needed to demonstrate to the patient how much weight they can bear through the affected limb.
WBAT	Weight bearing as tolerated (as pain or discomfort allows).
FWB	Full weight bearing.
TTWB	Toe-touch weight bearing. Foot touches the floor but no weight taken through the limb.

The choice of how much weight a patient can bear through their affected limb will depend on a number of factors. Factors such as pain, pathology, surgery, range of movement, muscle strength and the surgeon's instructions should all be taken into account. If patients are allowed to weight bear as tolerated, they will automatically restrict the amount of weight transferred to a limb after surgery and will increase the load as the bone and soft tissues heal (Koval et al., 1998). Regardless of the amount of weight bearing permitted, patients should be encouraged to walk with as close to a normal gait pattern as possible, i.e. normal heel–toe pattern and stride length, whilst avoiding hopping.

Types of walking aids

Crutches

Axillary crutches (Fig. 4.1)

The body weight must be transmitted through hands by extending elbows. These crutches are ideal for long-term use. Patients must be educated **not** to take unnecessary weight through the axilla. If left, this may cause damage to axillary vessels or nerves.

Elbow crutches (Fig. 4.2)

Some patients prefer crutches without the additional length of underarm support. Elbow crutches are suitable for younger patients as they are easier to manoeuvre and less cumbersome.

Gutter crutches

These are crutches with forearm support. They are used when patients are unable to take weight through the wrist and elbow. For example, if a patient sustains a fracture of the distal radius and is treated with a plaster of Paris, at the same time as a fractured neck of femur. Likewise patients

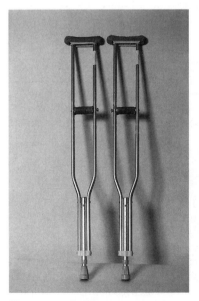
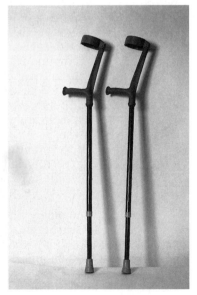

Figure 4.1. Axillary crutches.   **Figure 4.2.** Elbow crutches.

with instability and pain due to rheumatoid arthritis of the upper arm may benefit from the use of gutter crutches.

Frames

Frames offer a wide base of support while helping to lower the centre of gravity, therefore they are very stable. However, they are difficult to use on the stairs and a normal reciprocal gait pattern cannot be performed. There are a variety of different types of frames:

Basic frame

This is the most common frame used (Fig. 4.3). Some are made so that they can be folded and therefore transported easily.

Rollator frames (Fig. 4.4)

Some frames have wheels on the front two legs which make them easier to move forward. These may be useful for patients with weak upper extremities who find it easier to roll the frame forward rather than lift. There are rollator frames with four wheels on the market but these may be unsafe, depending on the client's abilities.

Gutter frame

This has the same principle as gutter crutches, allowing weight to be taken through the upper arm rather than the wrist.

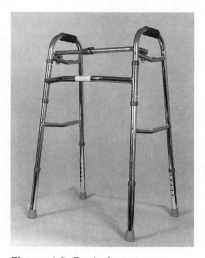

Figure 4.3. Basic frame.

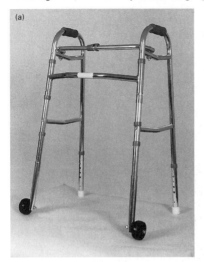 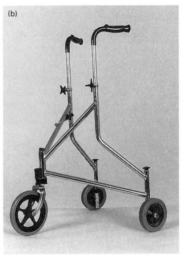

Figure 4.4. Two different types of rollator frame. (a) Folding frame with two front wheels. (b) Folding tri-frame with three wheels.

Single support

Walking stick

Walking sticks vary from the traditional wooden stick to lighter weight-adjustable aluminium models. A walking stick should be held in the opposite hand to the affected leg to gain maximum support. The walking stick and the affected leg should move together with the body weight being distributed between them as the unaffected leg moves forwards. Step length should be equal. Unilateral use of a walking stick can allow 15–25 per cent of a person's body weight to be supported (Ely and Smidt, 1977).

Quadrapod

This is a stick with four legs that provides more stability than a basic stick.

Measuring for walking aids

Where possible it is best to measure for any walking aid with the patient in a relaxed standing position wearing their usual footwear. This can be performed for most elective admissions when the patient is assessed pre-operatively. However, in other cases, patients may be measured for the first time post-operatively. In these cases, measurement should be performed in supine lying prior to standing the patient.

If the patient cannot lie completely supine for measurement, a temporary measure may require asking for the patient's height and adjusting the aid with respect to yourself.

Axillary crutches

The axilla height

Measure 5 cm (or three fingers' width) below the axilla to floor (20 cm out from the lateral heel). Figures 4.5 and 4.6 demonstrate measuring the length of the axillary portion of the crutches. Crutches that are too high will encourage the patient to lean on the axillary component and result in compression of the axillary nerve and vessels (Fig. 4.7).

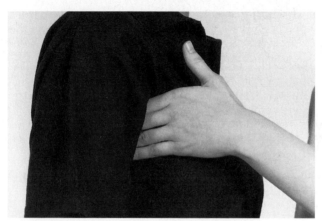

Figure 4.5. Measuring the axillary height.

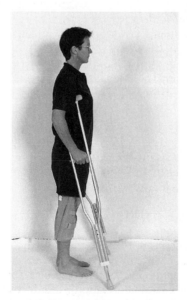

Figure 4.6. The correct position for axillary crutches. Note that the elbow is flexed at approximately 20°. The shoulders should be relaxed and the patient should not lean on the axilla component.

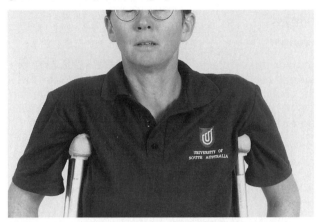

Figure 4.7. Demonstrates incorrect height of axillary crutches. If left this would lead to axillary artery and nerve compression.

The hand-piece height

With the elbow in 20° flexion, measure from the ulnar styloid to the floor (20 cm out from the lateral side of the heel).

Elbow crutches

The hand-piece height

With the elbow in 20° flexion, measure from the ulnar styloid to the floor (20 cm out from the lateral heel).

The elbow support should be adjusted so that it does not impinge on the extensor or flexor surface of the forearm during mobilization.

Frame/Stick

Measure from either the greater trochanter or the ulnar styloid with the elbow flexed no greater than 20° to the floor (20 cm away from the lateral heel).

Types of gait patterns

Gait patterns can be described as two, three or four point patterns. The points refer to the total number of discrete contacts the gait aid(s) and the lower limb(s) make with the supporting surface during a complete gait cycle. In general, the gait will become more stable as the number of points increases whilst also becoming increasingly slower.

Four point gait

This gait requires the use of bilateral aids such as two walking sticks. The pattern requires alternate and reciprocal advancement of the aid and the patient's opposite lower extremity, e.g. R crutch followed by the L leg. then L crutch followed by the R leg. The four point pattern provides a very stable base and requires low energy expenditure. However it is a very slow gait pattern. Most commonly this pattern is used when a patient suffers from a condition affecting both legs, for example, incomplete paraplegia.

Two point gait

This is similar to the four point pattern except that the aid and the opposite leg are advanced simultaneously, e.g. L crutch and R leg advanced simultaneously followed by simultaneous advancement of R crutch and L leg. This provides a faster more normal gait pattern than the four point pattern but there is some loss of stability. It also requires good coordination by the patient.

Three point gait

This allows for rapid ambulation but requires good upper body strength. Although it is a less stable pattern, it is probably the most commonly used pattern on an orthopaedic ward as it can be used for both NWB and PWB gait with all types of aids. It requires good upper body strength and good physical fitness. The pattern should be progressed from a step-to to a step-through pattern.

In the case of NWB, a modified three point gait can be used, i.e. when the affected leg is put forward but no weight is transferred through it. This is known as toe-touch weight bearing. This pattern requires a coordinated patient and means not putting any weight through the affected leg but the foot touches the floor, thus maintaining a normal gait pattern with heel strike and toe-off. Alternatively, the affected leg may be flexed at the knee so that it is not put to the floor.

Teaching PWB or NWB with a step-to gait pattern

The following points outline the instructions that the physiotherapist should give to the patient. A demonstration of the pattern by the physiotherapist should be performed first to ensure that the patient fully understands the concepts involved.

- Move both crutches forward, a good shoulder width apart.
- Bring the affected leg in line with the crutches and take a percentage of weight through it.
- Lean down through the hands and bring the good leg up to the crutches.

Figure 4.8 demonstrates a step-to gait pattern. Once safe with a step-to-gait pattern the patient should be progressed to a step-through pattern

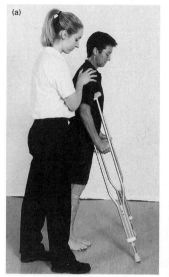 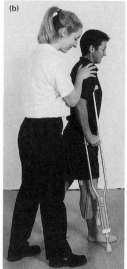 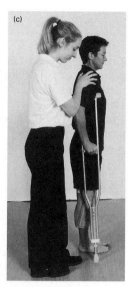

Figure 4.8. (a–c) Step to three point gait pattern with axillary crutches. Note that the physiotherapist is standing on the affected side and slightly behind the patient.

whereby the unaffected leg is taken past the crutches and has a normal stride length (Fig. 4.9).

When this is taught in the NWB situation there is a tendency, especially for nervous patients, to hop on the 'good' leg and merely use crutches for balance. This is not only very unstable but is also very tiring to maintain. The patient must be taught to use a correct pattern and to toe-touch if permitted.

Mobilization following prolonged bed rest

Prolonged bed rest is usually required for patients sustaining multiple trauma with severe bilateral lower leg fractures and/or pelvic fractures. Prolonged bed rest will result in postural hypotension, lack of balance, weakness, decreased flexibility, reduced coordination and lack of confidence of the patient. Due to these factors mobilization will require a slow yet sustained rehabilitation effort. To accustom the patient to changes in blood pressure it is often necessary to transfer the patient to a tilt bed. A tilt table can be moved through varying degrees, from the horizontal, working towards the upright vertical position. This process may take from 2–7 days as it is likely that patients will experience nausea and dizziness. If weight bearing is to be restricted it may be necessary to monitor by placing a set of scales under one foot and a leveller under the other to instruct the patient on how much weight they can bear. If PWB is achieved, the patient may move from lie to sit and be taught bed

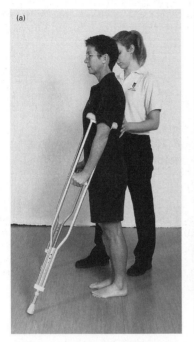

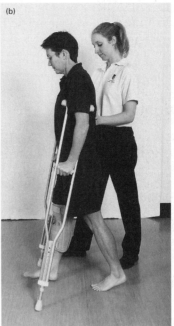

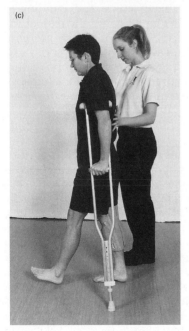

Figure 4.9. (a–c) Step through three point gait pattern.

to chair transfers. When moving from sit to stand it will be necessary to have one or two assistants to support the patient and reassure them. The first stages of walking may be achieved using a gutter frame with which the patient can support themselves through their upper body. Once walking has been mastered with this aid, the patient may change to elbow or axillary crutches and then gradually reduce the use of these until FWB is achieved.

Functional activities

Before any patient returns to their home environment with a walking aid, it is imperative that the physiotherapist ensures that they are functionally independent with the gait aid. Patients may need to be able to get out of bed, ascend or descend steps and stairs, walk backwards or sideways and turn around. The physiotherapist should ascertain which functional abilities will be required by the patient and ensure that the patient is safe and competent in performing these activities before returning home. It is important to be aware of any functional restrictions that may have been imposed by the surgeon. Precautions after THR are commonly imposed to reduce the incidence of post-operative dislocation and may include restrictions of flexion and rotation.

Sitting and standing

Each patient must be taught how to achieve sitting and standing safely and independently using their aid(s). Before standing the patient should shuffle forward in the chair. This brings the centre of gravity nearer to the base of support and facilitates standing. Patients will often find it easier if they place the foot of the unaffected leg as far back as possible. This provides a better push off from the unaffected and presumably stronger leg. If both lower extremities are affected then the foot of the dominant leg is often put behind. Whilst assisting the patient, the physiotherapist should always stand on the affected side as protection in the event that the patient loses balance.

Immediately following a THR patients should avoid bending forward (restrict hip flexion) and keep both feet and knees pointing forward (neutral hip rotation) when they get up from a sitting position.

Patients must be taught to use the strength in their upper extremities to assist the stand. They should push simultaneously on the arms of the chair as they lean their body weight forward. When using a frame, patients must not pull on the frame as they stand because again this is unstable and the frame will invariably topple over. They should place their hands on the frame only when they have reached the standing position.

With crutches, the patient has two choices, either (1) to push up on the arms of a chair, and then retrieve crutches, or (2) push up with one hand (on the affected side) on the arm of a chair and the other hand on the hand grips of the crutches which have been placed together. The crutches should be held on the unaffected side (Fig. 4.10). Once the patient is standing the crutches can then be transferred.

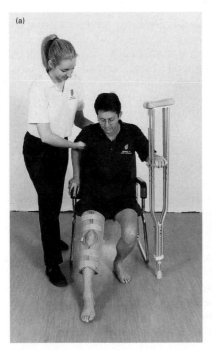 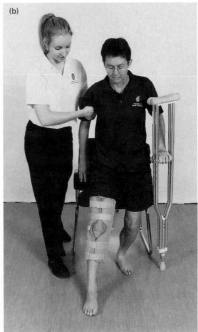

Figure 4.10. (a, b) Standing from a chair using axillary crutches. Physiotherapist guides from the affected side.

Sitting down in chair

When sitting back down in a chair the patient should be instructed to walk backwards until they can feel the front of the seat on the back of their legs. The crutches should then be transferred to one hand, holding them at the hand grip (on the unaffected side). Then the patient should lean forwards, bend the unaffected leg to sit, using their free hand on the seat or armrest of the chair. The physiotherapist should always investigate whether the chair is safe (i.e. brakes on) and prevent it from moving with their foot if necessary. Support of the affected leg may also be required whilst the patient sits down.

Ascending and descending stairs

Before any patient is discharged from hospital it is important that they are taught how to negotiate stairs with their walking aid. This is imperative if the patient has stairs or steps in their home. Stairs should be only attempted if the patient has good balance, strength and trunk control. It is generally only feasible to achieve stair climbing with crutches or walking sticks. Patients requiring the use of a frame will be too unsteady to attempt stairs in addition to the frame being too cumbersome. However, it may be necessary to teach the patient how to negotiate a single step as many homes have some sort of step. In this instance the same principles apply that are described below.

When ascending or descending stairs, the affected leg and gait aid should travel together. The physiotherapist should always stand below the patient in the event that the patient loses their balance. When ascending the stairs, the physiotherapist should therefore stand behind and below the patient and when descending, the physiotherapist is in front and below the patient. The patient should be supported by the physiotherapist at waist height where necessary. When the patient requires bilateral crutches then there are two ways that they can master stairs. The patient can either use the crutches bilaterally or, if there is a banister, then the patient can place the crutch closest to the banister horizontally along the hand grip of the crutch furthest away from the banister. This will allow the patient to use the banister for support.

Instructions

Ascending stairs (Fig. 4.11)
Step up as close to the stairs as possible.
Place the unaffected leg on the first step.
Put your weight through and straighten the unaffected leg.
Lift the crutches and affected leg to the same step as the 'good' leg.

Descending stairs (Fig. 4.12)
Stand close to edge of the step.
Place the crutches and affected leg down to step below.
Bend the good leg and slowly let the affected leg and the crutches reach the step below.
Lean through the crutches to lower good leg to the same step as the affected leg.

The much loved and well used expression 'Good leg up to heaven and bad leg down to hell' helps patients and physiotherapists alike remember the sequence for ascending and descending stairs.

Occupational health and safety when teaching the use of walking aids

1. Check any rubber tips (ferules) for wear and safe design. Replace any rounded or shiny rubber tips which may not grip well and therefore slip easily.
2. Warn the patient about water on the floor, as this allows rubber tips to slip.
3. Provide regular maintenance of all equipment, e.g. check that screws and bolts in crutches are firmly secured.
4. Teach the patient a gait that gives as large and wide a base as possible.
5. Teach the patient to maintain a large base when standing still (usually stand with crutches slightly ahead of the feet).

(a)

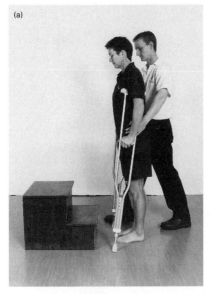

(b)

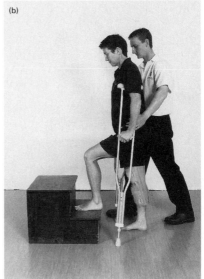

(c)

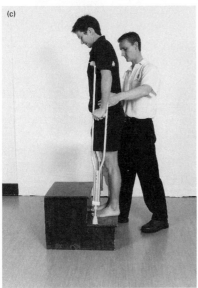

Figure 4.11. (a–c) Ascending stairs.

6. When standing up with a frame, the patient must be instructed to push up on the arms of the chair and must not pull on the frame.
7. At all times the physiotherapist must be positioned to prevent falls, usually standing to the side and slightly behind the affected side.
8. Prior to discharge from hospital each patient should be independent in getting up from a chair; walking forwards, backwards and sideways; turning around; stairs; and sitting.

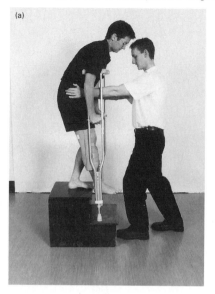

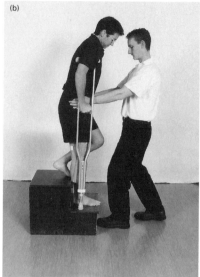

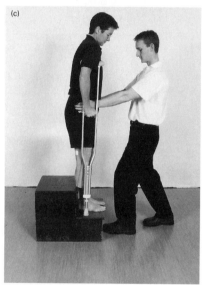

Figure 4.12. (a–c) Descending stairs.

Gait education – precautions

- Ensure that the patient is wearing appropriate footwear. Do not allow the patient to wear loose-fitting shoes when ambulating. Never mobilize a patient with just their socks on. In these instances the patient may be unsteady or at risk of slipping. It is best to mobilize a patient in well-fitting shoes with good grip or no shoes at all.

- During ambulation, frequently monitor and observe the patient's general appearance and alertness, e.g. sudden pallor. Keep a chair close by or have a colleague assisting if you are concerned about a patient.
- At all times when mobilizing a patient, the physiotherapist must stay alert. The physiotherapist should not become complacent or distracted in the event that the patient may fall, faint or stumble. The physiotherapist should stand to the side and slightly behind the patient.
- The patient should never be left unattended while standing or sitting on the edge of the bed.
- Protect any attachments such as an IV line, catheters and other appliances whilst ambulating and transferring.
- Be aware of any special precautions, e.g. post THR avoid flexion over 90° when transferring.
- Before ambulating, the physiotherapist should make sure that the area is safe. Any potential hazards, such as tables and chairs or water on the floor must be removed.

Recording transfer and gait retraining techniques

Accurate recording of the amount of assistance required by the patient during transfer or gait retraining techniques is very important. Other health professionals required to lift or transfer patients will need an indication of the support required by the patient. Therefore the following abbreviations are used in case notes for recording the amount of assistance required by the patient.

LA = light assist.
MA = moderate assist.
HA = heavy assist.
SB = standby.

Example
Mobilized PWB × 2 LA means mobilized the patient partial weight bearing with two light assists.

References

Ely, D. D. and Smidt, G. L. (1977). Effect of cane on variables of gait for patients with hip disorders. *Physical Therapy*, **57**, 507–512.

Koval, K. J., Sala, D. A., Kummer, F. J. and Zuckerman, J. D. (1998). Postoperative weight-bearing after a fracture of the femoral neck or an intertrochanteric fracture. *J. Bone Joint Surg.*, **80A**, 352–364.

Simpson, C. and Pirrie, L. (1991). Walking aids – a survey of suitability and supply. *Physiotherapy*, **77**, 231–234.

CHAPTER 5

Transfer and lifting techniques

The ability to assist with the movement of patients is an important role of physiotherapists in any healthcare setting. As a team member trained in the biomechanics of posture and movement, physiotherapists are often called upon to give advice and education on safe and effective transfers and lifting to other staff members. In addition, following orthopaedic surgery, patients generally require independence in safe transfer techniques prior to discharge to their home environment. This chapter covers key principles involved in transfer and lifting techniques. Examples of common techniques used in a general orthopaedic ward are also included.

Definitions

Manual handling

This term is used to describe any activity which requires the use of force by a therapist to lower, pull, carry or move a patient or piece of equipment.

Lifting

Lifting involves a therapist moving or raising a patient or piece of equipment where vertical displacement is the main component. The therapist(s) bears most of the weight.

Transfer

Transferring a patient involves techniques that move a patient horizontally, where the patient assists, so that only a percentage of the weight is borne by the therapist(s).

Hospital policy

The incidence of injury to healthcare workers has been shown to be approximately 30 per cent higher than in any other industry (Foley and Cole, 1995). Holder et al. (1999) demonstrated that 32 per cent of physiotherapists reported sustaining a musculoskeletal injury in the course of their work, with the highest prevalence of injury being the low back. Manual handling has been shown to be the commonest mechanism of injury (Knibbe and Friele, 1996). To minimize the potential risk of musculoskeletal injury to healthcare workers, hospitals and governments have implemented Occupational Health and Safety policies and manual handling codes. Prior to working in any hospital it is therefore important that the physiotherapist become familiar and comply with the policy of their workplace.

Many hospitals in Australia have recently implemented, what has been given the nomenclature, 'no lifting' or 'zero lifting' policies. In general, these policies require that lifting of patients be eliminated in all but exceptional or life-threatening situations. Indeed some policies suggest that manual handling should only continue if it does not involve lifting most or all of a patient's weight. In the clinical setting this means that patients who can assist in their transfer should be encouraged and, where possible, be taught to do so. When patients are unable to assist, specialist equipment, such as hydraulic hoists and other lifting devices/equipment, should be utilized to minimize unnecessary strain on the worker. Hospitals with 'no lifting' policies, therefore, must have appropriate equipment available to assist all staff with transferring and lifting patients. Not all hospitals have assumed this 'no lifting' policy, therefore it is still important that physiotherapists have effective means to both transfer and lift patients.

Transfers

A transfer is the safe and effective movement of a person from one surface or location to another or from one position to another (Pierson, 1994). Transfer techniques range from assisting a patient to a better position in bed to helping someone out of bed.

Transfers can be classified as:

Independent   Patient is safe, efficient and effective without needing assistance.

Dependent   Patient requires physical assistance of one or more persons or piece of equipment.

Indirect assistance   Patient only requires indirect assistance, such as standby assistance (SA), usually only until they have gained confidence.

Preparation for transfer

Adequate preparation is required prior to performing any transfer technique. Preparation should always include a comprehensive patient assessment, as well as attending to environmental and personnel needs. Any equipment to be used during the transfer should also be prepared.

A comprehensive assessment of each patient will help ascertain the capabilities and limitations of each patient. The assessment should include examination of the patient for subjective and objective information. This will include their prior abilities and more detailed objective measures such as muscle strength. Further relevant information should also be gained from the case notes, e.g. patient compliance with therapy, mental status, blood gas levels.

From this information the physiotherapist will be able to determine how much assistance will be required. Extra personnel or mechanical aids, such as overhead pulleys, may be utilized depending on the patient's capabilities and their post-operative plan with regard to any specific contraindications or precautions. Following this the physiotherapist should arrange the environment. Furniture may have to be moved to allow a clear space. Any additional hazards, such as water on the floor, should be dealt with as necessary. All equipment should also be examined. For instance, ensuring that the wheel brakes have been applied in equipment such as wheelchairs or beds.

General principles governing transfers

There are several principles that should be adhered to when performing any lift or transfer of a patient. Applying these principles will ensure a safe and effective outcome.

Explanation and reassurance

A clear and concise explanation of the lift or transfer must be given to the patient. Physiotherapists working on orthopaedic wards are often the first people to transfer or move the conscious patient. Patients are likely to be in some degree of pain as well as being anxious about what is happening. An explanation of what to expect will help to alleviate this anxiety and fear. If the patient is required to assist in the transfer, it is often better to get them to repeat back to the physiotherapist what is required after the explanation. This will ensure that the patient fully comprehends. Simply asking if they understand will usually obtain an affirmative response whether the patient understands or not.

Patient preparation

The patient should then be physically prepared for the transfer. This may involve helping them to dress or put on shoes and socks. Avoid poor fitting trousers and hospital gowns that do not tie up properly. Loose-fitting shoes, slippers or socks should also not be worn when standing or walking the patient as this may result in the patient slipping or tripping. Bare feet or a pair of well-fitting shoes are preferable. Any patient attachments, such as wound drains, must be organized so that they do not become caught or entangled during the transfer.

Physiotherapist position during the transfer

When performing the transfer, the physiotherapist(s) should maintain a broad stable base whilst keeping the load as close to them as possible. A good grip is also important. The physiotherapist's knees should be bent and the spinal curves maintained during the transfer. Maintaining a good spinal posture and bracing of the abdominal muscles prior to lifting will help prevent any spinal injuries during lifting. Transference of the physiotherapist's body weight, extension of the knees and use of the patient's momentum should help achieve any transfer.

Instruction

The physiotherapist should instruct the patient and any other helpers about when to start the lift. Most commonly the verbal instructions are: 'On the word lift, after three ... one, two, three ... lift.'

Precautions following orthopaedic surgery

Total hip replacement

Following a total hip replacement by a posterior approach (see Chapter 6, page 84), there is a risk of dislocation if the hip is forced into flexion, internal rotation and adduction. In fact, some surgeons do not allow patients to sit until 47 days after the surgery. In these instances, patients must be transferred out of bed without the operated leg moving into flexion, internal rotation and adduction. The technique used to transfer a patient with a THR out of bed on the first post-operative day is described in Chapter 6, page 87.

Spinal surgery

Following some spinal surgery, for example a spinal fusion, patients may have to avoid lumbar flexion and rotation. Furthermore, any movement of the spine may cause the patient discomfort. Therefore log rolling must be taught to the patient so that the spine is not forced into a flexion or rotation. Log rolling requires moving the spine as one.

Bed mobility

Bed mobility transfers are important, particularly if a patient has to stay on bed rest for a prolonged period. The use of ORIF allows most patients to be mobilized early, thus minimizing the deleterious effects of prolonged bed rest. However, there are still a few instances where bed rest for an extended period may be required, e.g. patients with multiple lower limb trauma. In these instances, teaching the patient how to move about in bed will promote independence, prevent pressure areas and joint contractures.

Pressure sores are one of the leading causes of orthopaedic patient morbidity and mortality. Moreover, the development of a pressure sore will result in a considerable increase in the duration and cost of a patient's length of stay in hospital. In addition, most pressure sores are preventable with regular and thorough pressure area care. This is normally under the care of the nursing staff although all professionals involved in direct patient care should be aware of this problem.

Moving across the bed (side to side)

If the patient is unable to sit, e.g. following a THR

First the patient should be instructed to flex their non-operated leg. In this half crook-lying position, their hands can then be placed either on the overhead hook (if available) or at the side of their hips (Fig. 5.1). The physiotherapist should stand on the side the patient is moving towards. The physiotherapist can assist by helping the patient's pelvis across by placing a hand (or two) under their pelvis and leaning backwards. The patient then moves their shoulders across. If there is no overhead assistance, but there are two helpers, they can provide a support for the patient by leaning towards each other and each bracing a hand on the other's shoulder.

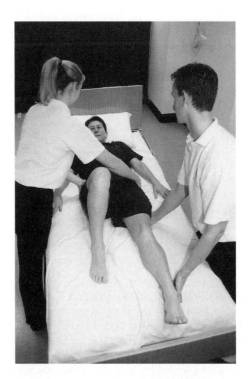

Figure 5.1. Moving sideways across the bed. The physiotherapist controlling the transfer stands on the side that the patient is moving to whilst the other physiotherapist supports the affected leg.

If the patient is able to sit and can manage a long sitting position

In this instance, moving across in bed should be relatively easy, particularly for the younger or fitter patient. The patient flexes their unaffected leg whilst in the long sitting position (Fig. 5.2). The patient should push into the bed with their hands and unaffected leg whilst lifting their pelvis sideways. The physiotherapist supports the affected leg when and if necessary. This technique is not suitable following hip surgery.

Rolling in bed

Teaching this manoeuvre is important following spinal surgery where flexion of the spine may not be allowed. The physiotherapist should stand on the side of the bed that the patient is rolling towards. The patient should then flex both knees to the crook-lying position. The patient grasps their hands together and places them out in front of themselves. The patient should be instructed to move the spine as one, e.g. 'roll over like a log by keeping your spine straight'. Slowly they should log roll over with the physiotherapist supporting and directing from the hip and shoulder.

From this side-lying position the physiotherapist can then assist the patient into a sitting position, again taking care not to flex or rotate the spine.

Sitting up in bed

Depending on the ability and strength of the patient this may require one or two physiotherapists. The physiotherapist(s) should stand facing the head end of the bed. A stride-stance position should be adopted with the outside foot at the patient's mid-thorax level whilst the inside foot is level with the patient's mid-thigh region. The arm closer to the foot of the bed

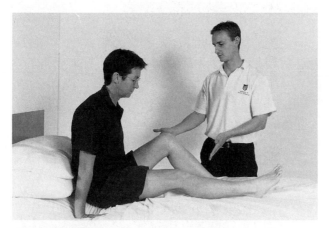

Figure 5.2. Moving across the bed independently in the long sitting position.

passes under the patient's arm to hold onto the scapula posteriorly. The other arm supports the patient's head if necessary or can be positioned over the scapula more medially. The patient's elbows should be in flexion with their hand(s) on the back of the physiotherapist(s) upper arms. The physiotherapist(s) should then assist the patient to the sitting position by leaning their body weight back (Fig. 5.3).

Moving up the bed

Assistance available from the patient

Assist the patient into a sitting position. The unaffected leg should be flexed so that the patient can use it to propel themselves up the bed. The patient can then either push down on the bed with their hands or grab hold of the overhead monkey bar. The physiotherapist should support the patient near the buttock fold. This may require two physiotherapists particularly if the operated leg requires support during the transfer.

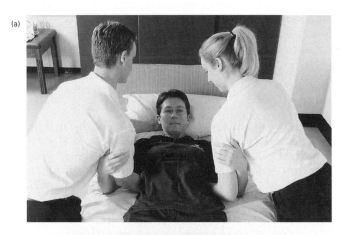

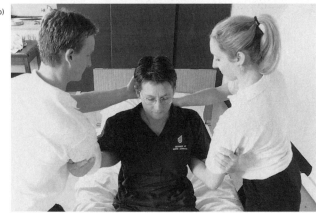

Figure 5.3. (a, b) Sitting the patient up in bed.

Lifting techniques

Where the patient is unable to assist, it may be necessary to perform a lift. If the patient is in a supine position and needs to be moved up the bed, then a draw sheet or similar device can be used to lift the patient. At least two people and in some circumstances four or five assistants may be required depending on the weight and ability of the patient. Each lifter should be in the stride stance on either side of the bed. The draw sheet should be rolled in as far towards the patient as possible. The draw sheet should then be grasped firmly at the level of the patient's knees and lower back. The patient should cross their arms across their chest (Fig. 5.4). If the patient can assist they should be asked to lift their head off the bed and to tuck their chin into their chest. If this is not possible an extra assistant may be required to support the head and neck during the lift. On the pre-arranged instruction the patient can be transferred up or down the bed. Sliding sheets may also be used in the same manner. With these the patient is slid up the bed rather than lifted.

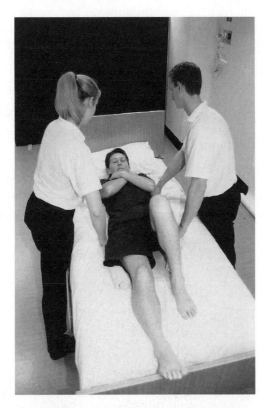

Figure 5.4. Using a draw sheet to transfer the patient up the bed. The patient is assisting with the transfer by pushing with the left leg.

Shoulder lift

The shoulder lift can be used in a variety of situations but is not possible for patients who have undergone shoulder surgery or who have shoulder joint pathology, e.g. for a patient with rheumatoid arthritis (RA) affecting the shoulder. This is also not a good lift for a patient who has undergone a THR as it requires too much hip flexion. The amount of hip flexion will be painful and risk dislocation.

This transfer helps to move the patient back in the bed so is useful for sitting up patients who have slipped down the bed. Two physiotherapists are required for this transfer.

The physiotherapists should be on opposite sides of the bed, each in stride stance facing the head end of the bed. Each back foot should be approximately at the level of the patient's buttocks whilst the front foot should be positioned comfortably forwards (Fig. 5.5).

The physiotherapists should reach under the client's upper thighs with a monkey or forearm grip of the arm closest to the bed (Fig. 5.6). The front arm can either be placed on the bed or on the patient's scapula if they are unsteady in a sitting position. In the lifting position the patient's arms should rest down each of the physiotherapists' backs (Fig. 5.7). The patient should be instructed to lean down through their arms onto the physiotherapist, i.e. adduct their arms. On the prearranged instruction the physiotherapists should transfer the patient back up the bed by leaning on

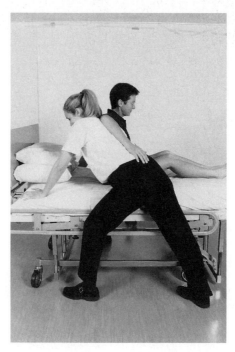

Figure 5.5. Physiotherapist in stride stance position.

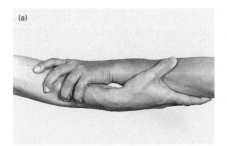
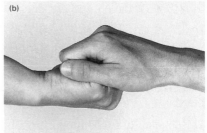

Figure 5.6. (a) Forearm grasp. (b) Monkey grip.

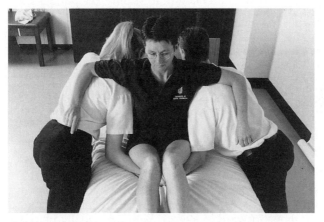

Figure 5.7. Position for shoulder lift. Patient's arms
resting along the physiotherapists' backs

the free arm, straightening their knees, and transferring weight to the
forward position leg.

This lift can be modified if the patient has had shoulder surgery and
cannot move one arm. The same lift is achieved but with the affected arm
maintained in a sling whilst the unaffected arm is placed along the back of
one physiotherapist.

Equipment

There are various different pieces of equipment that can be used to assist
with the transfer of lifting of patients. When required to use equipment for
lifting, the following guidelines should be followed (Dean and Timbs,
1997):

- All physiotherapists should be trained in the correct use of the
  equipment.
- Equipment is regularly maintained.

- Use of the equipment does reduce the effort required by the lifters.
- Use of equipment is safe for both the physiotherapists and the patient.
- Use of equipment allows the patient to assist as much as possible.

Overhead bar (sometimes known as self-help poles or monkey bars)

This is usually suspended from a pole attached to the frame at the head of the bed. This can be used to obtain independent bed mobility or to assist with transfer techniques. Overhead bars are only useful for patients with good upper limb strength and range of motion. The height of the bar must be correct to be of maximum benefit. In supine, the patient should be able to grip the bar, with their elbows slightly flexed.

Slide sheet (also known as a 'slippery sam')

This is a sheet of frictionless shiny material rather like sail-cloth that can be used to assist moving patients in bed. Rather than lifting a patient, with the cloth underneath, it can be used to slide the patient up or down the bed or to roll the patient.

Transfer bands and belts

A variety of commercially designed different bands or belts are available that can be used to assist with transfers. Firm bands with two handles at either end for the lifter to grasp can be used to help patients to stand, sit up in bed or move forward in a chair. Belts are usually placed around the patient's waist with the physiotherapist using the belt to pull on during the transfer.

Slide board

This is a rectangular piece of highly polished timber, again which reduces friction. The timber can be used to bridge the gap between two beds or chairs so that the patient can be slid across the board.

Pivot or swivel board

This consists of two discs of wood between which are ball bearings. This allows one disk to rotate easily on the other. These are most commonly used to transfer a patient who is unable to move their feet from one sitting position to another. For example, moving a patient from sitting on the edge of a bed to a wheelchair. A strap may need to be used in conjunction with the pivot board.

Hydraulic lifting machines

The use of large hydraulic lifting machines will help eliminate lifting but still requires the transfer of the patient (Fig. 5.8).

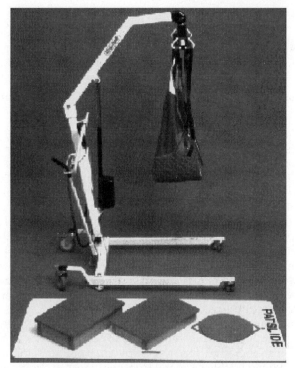

Figure 5.8. Type of mechanical hoist (reproduced with permission from Smith and Nephew).

References

Dean, P. and Timbs, P. (1997). *The Manual Handling Instruction Book*. South Australia. ISBN 0 9587176 2 1.

Foley, G. and Cole, B. (1995). *Occupational Health and Safety Performance Overviews*. Selected Industries Issue No 7. Worksafe Australia. Australian Government Publishing.

Holder, N. L., Clark, H. A., DiBlasio, J. M., Hughes, C. L. et al. (1999). Cause, prevalence, and response to occupation musculoskeletal injuries reported by physical therapists and physical therapist assistants. *Physical Therapy*, **79**, 642–652.

Knibbe, J. J. and Friele, R. D. (1996). Prevalence of low back pain and characteristics of the physical workload of community nurses. *Ergonomics*, **39**, 186–198.

Pierson, F. M. (1994). *Principles and Techniques of Patient Care*. WB Saunders Company.

CHAPTER 6

Hip surgery

The hip joint is one of the most important joints of the body, providing stability for the transmission of the body weight during normal gait whilst allowing mobility for functional activities of daily living, such as sitting down and climbing stairs. Thus the joint is a 'ball and socket' joint constructed for stability whilst permitting a large range of movement. Surgery to the hip joint tends to fall into two categories: those for younger patients with sequelae of paediatric hip conditions and those for older patients with fractures, osteoarthritis or osteoporosis. Of this group the most common surgeries are total hip replacement (THR) and fracture fixation, such as dynamic hip screws (DHS) for fractures of the neck of femur. The post-operative physiotherapy management following these surgical procedures is very similar except that there are some precautions that need to be adhered to following THR.

Total hip replacement

Definitions

Hip joint	A ball and socket joint formed by the head of the femur and the acetabulum.
THR	A total hip replacement is an artificial joint where both the femoral and acetabular sides of the hip joint are replaced. The femoral implant is placed within the medullary canal of the femur and proximally has a small diameter head that articulates with a corresponding socket that is fixed into the acetabulum (Fig. 6.1).
Cemented THR	The femoral and acetabular components are both inserted with bone cement (poly-methyl-methacrylate, PMMA) that bonds the implant to the prepared bone of the acetabulum and femoral medullary canal (Fig. 6.2). This provides immediate solid fixation of the THR to the bone. Most commonly used in elderly patients.

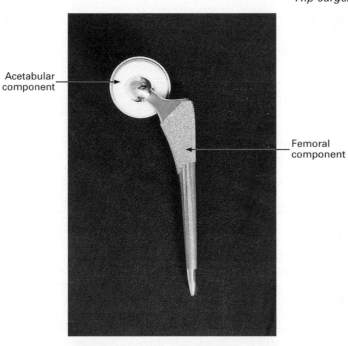

Acetabular component

Femoral component

Figure 6.1. Component parts for a THR.

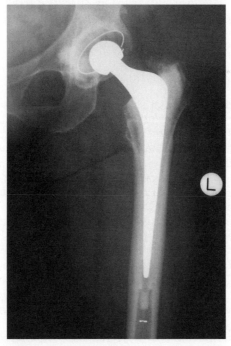

Figure 6.2. Antero-posterior radiograph of a cemented THR in situ.

Cementless THR	The femoral and acetabular components are both inserted without bone cement. The THR components have a porous texture that allows the in-growth of bone onto the surface of the implant. Immediate fixation is provided by an interference fit of the component into the prepared bone. This is often achieved by implanting a component that is 1–2 mm larger than the prepared acetabulum or femoral canal.
Hybrid THR	A THR where one implant, usually the femoral stem, is cemented and the acetabular cup is cementless. This combination is the most common type of THR used in Australia.
Revision THR	Any subsequent operation that is performed due to loosening, infection, dislocation, fracture or other causes of implant failure of the first or primary THR.
Excision arthroplasty	This is an operation that involves complete resection of the hip joint leaving a gap that fills with fibrous tissue. The end result is a joint with reduced pain but which is functionally second rate. The operation is also known as a Girdlestone procedure and is rarely performed these days due to the success of THR and revision surgery. A Girdlestone procedure would only be performed as a last resort salvage procedure for severe infection after THR.

Outcomes of THR

Total hip replacement is perhaps one of the most successful and common surgical procedures of the twentieth century. The success of THR surgery has been strongly supported by long-term follow-up studies (10–20 years) with the prosthetic survival rate reported to be approximately 90 per cent (Franzen et al., 1997; Malchau and Herberts, 1998). In addition to this, long-term follow up has demonstrated that 90 per cent of patients achieve successful clinical outcomes in terms of pain relief and improvements in function (O'Boyle et al., 1992; Rorebeck et al., 1994). More recently studies have demonstrated immediate and substantial improvements in the pain, functional abilities and overall health-related quality of life (Gogia et al., 1994; Rissanen et al., 1996). THR surgery has also been shown to be a highly cost-effective procedure for the community (Bourne and Kim, 1998; NHS Centre for Reviews and Dissemination, 1996). The long-term success is dependent on the type of implant used, the surgical technique and several patient factors including obesity, activity levels and age of patient (Swedish Hip Registry).

Excellent long-term results are only available for several THRs which all have cemented metal femoral stems, metal femoral heads and cemented all-polyethylene acetabular cups, e.g. Charnley hip replacement

(Wroblewski and Siney, 1993). There are many other types of THR available. Each are made with variations in design and materials. Newer designs and materials which incorporate cementless fixation, hydroxy-apatite coatings and ceramic bearing surfaces should not be regarded as better until they have been proved in long-term studies (Fender et al., 1999; Muirhead-Allwood, 1998).

Indications

Patients who are candidates for total hip replacement are those who have disabling pain and functional limitation of the hip despite a trial of adequate conservative therapy (drug therapy, physiotherapy). Of the multiple causes of pain in the hip, the ones most likely to necessitate the need for a total joint replacement are:

- Primary osteoarthritis (OA). Prevalence studies indicate that osteoarthritis is the most common hip disorder facing the elderly. Figure 6.3 demonstrates osteoarthritis of the hip. Primary OA may include patients with unrecognized or untreated acetabular dysplasia.
- Secondary OA. This may be due to childhood hip disorders including developmental dysplasia of the hip, Legg–Calve–Perthes disease (LCPD) and slipped capital femoral epiphysis (SCFE). Secondary

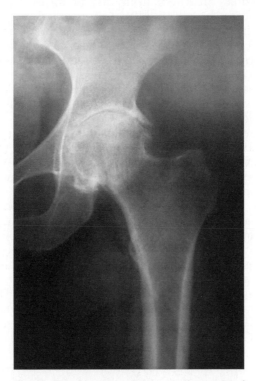

Figure 6.3. Antero-posterior radiograph of the hip demonstrating OA.

OA may also develop following severe trauma or fractures around the hip joint.

- Following fracture of the neck of femur.
- Avascular necrosis (AVN) of the femoral head.
- Rheumatoid arthritis (RA).
- Benign and malignant tumours – the use of a THR in patients with malignant tumour is weighed up against their life expectancy and quality of life.

The indications for revision arthroplasty are aseptic loosening due to mechanical failure of the primary (first) implant or as a response to wear debris, recurrent dislocation due to implant malposition or muscle imbalance, infection, periprosthetic fracture of the femur or acetabulum and implant breakage.

Revision hip replacement is a much more technically demanding operation and usually requires a longer hospital stay with a higher complication rate. Patients undergoing revision surgery gain similar improvements in pain and quality of life; however, long-term functional outcomes are not as good as primary procedures (Robinson et al., 1999).

Hospital requirements

Pre-admission clinics are a recent introduction for elective THR surgery aimed at improving the quality of patient care and reduce the average length of stay in hospital. Patients are seen in a pre-admission clinic approximately 4 weeks prior to surgery where they are assessed for surgery by an anaesthetist and pre-operative investigations are taken.

Patients are encouraged to donate their own blood that can be returned to the patient post-operatively. This reduces the need for blood to be taken from a blood bank, which in turn reduces the risk of transfusion related reactions and blood-borne infections.

The medical and physiotherapy staff should educate the patient regarding the operation and post-operative rehabilitation. Information regarding the expectations following surgery, pain relief and mobilization are explained. The patient's discharge plan and home requirements are formulated. Pre-operative education programmes, such as instructive pamphlets and videos, are also extremely useful for patients. Indeed, patients who have received pre-operative education have been shown to be less anxious at the time of hospital admission and at discharge, are more likely to have practised physiotherapy exercises prior to hospitalization and require less physiotherapy while in hospital (Butler et al., 1996). As with all elective procedures, the physiotherapy pre-operative assessment should be performed in the SOAP format. This will allow identification of patients who may require further assistance post-operatively. The SOAP assessment should include the following:

Subjective

Subjective factors that may impact on the patient's post-operative recovery and eventual discharge should be ascertained. In particular:

- Determination of the patient's social situation, e.g. whether an able-bodied carer is in the home or whether social services will be needed.
- Determination of the accessibility of the home environment, e.g. steps, stairs, access to toilet, shower and bath.
- Present mobilization status.
- Present respiratory function.
- Current health status including the identification of any co-morbid conditions that may affect the patient's outcome.

Objective

- Respiratory function.
- Range of movement and strength of other limbs.
- Strength and range of movement (ROM) of affected hip.
- Gait assessment.
- Leg length discrepancy.
- Trendelenburg's test.

Assessment

- Any factors that may affect the patient's outcome should be noted.

Plan

- Implement and teach patient post-operative exercise programme.
- Teach mobilization technique required post-operatively including use of aids such as a frame or crutches.
- Educate and advise regarding the hospital stay and expected length of recovery.
- Education regarding 'Dos and Don'ts' following surgery and any adaptations required for the patient's home environment.

Surgical anatomy and treatment

Access to the hip joint to perform THR is most commonly performed by either a posterior or lateral approach to the hip joint. The patient is placed in a lateral position with the affected hip uppermost. Specialized approaches for revision and difficult primary THR have been described and often involve osteotomy of the greater trochanter and reattachment with wires or cables (Campbell et al., 1998).

The posterior approach to the hip joint is made through a curved incision of 15–20 cm based over the posterior aspect of the greater trochanter. The superficial dissection is through the fascia lata and proximally the gluteus maximus is split in the line of its fibres. The sciatic nerve emerges from the greater sciatic notch, lying close to the posterior acetabular wall and is in danger throughout the operation. The deep dissection involves detaching the short rotators of the hip joint (piriformis, the gemelli, obturator internus, and quadratus femoris) from the proximal femur.

The hip capsule is then exposed and can be removed. The hip is then dislocated posteriorly by flexion, adduction and internal rotation.

The posterior approach provides an excellent exposure of the hip for primary and revision THR but has a higher rate of dislocation than the direct lateral approach. This is due to removing the posterior capsule, dividing the short external rotators and the position of the acetabular cup. This places the hip at risk of dislocation when the hip is flexed and internally rotated.

The lateral approach to the hip joint is made through a straight incision of 15 cm over the greater trochanter. The superficial dissection is through fascia lata and tensor fascia lata. The deep dissection involves detaching the part of the gluteus medius, minimus and vastus lateralis from the greater trochanter. The superior gluteal nerve is at risk when splitting the gluteus medius greater than 5 cm above the level of the greater trochanter. The hip capsule is then exposed and can be removed. The hip is then dislocated anteriorly by adduction, extension and external rotation.

The lateral approach may result in a Trendelenburg gait due to weakness of the hip abductor mechanism. This may be due to the dissection of the muscles or due to damage to the superior gluteal nerve with resultant nerve palsy. This may be present up to 12 months after surgery.

After exposure of the hip joint, the femoral neck is cut at a level proximal to the lesser trochanter. The acetabulum is prepared by removing all remaining cartilage and diseased bone and then an acetabular component is inserted. The ideal position is 40° of inclination and 15° of anteversion. The femur is then prepared and a femoral component is inserted with 10° of anteversion and in the longitudinal axis of the femur. The femoral component is placed so that the centre of the head is at the same level as the top of the greater trochanter. Stability, soft tissue tension and leg lengths are assessed and the components can be adjusted if required. An anatomical repair of all muscles and tissues is performed and the wound sutured.

Revision THR surgery is more complex than primary THR and may take between 2 and 6 hours. Problems facing the surgeon include removing the implants, osteolysis (bone loss around the components), fracture and abnormal anatomy. Revision surgery is different for all cases and the post-operative plan will vary with many patients.

Radiology

Plain radiography of the hip joints and femurs are taken pre-operatively and routinely include an antero-posterior (A-P) view of the pelvis and lateral view of the hip joint. The radiographs are used to diagnose pathology affecting the hip joint and to plan the surgical procedure. Plastic templates are used to determine the correct size of implants that will restore the anatomy of the hip joint and result in equal leg lengths.

Post-operatively the THR is assessed with plain radiography and an A-P and lateral view are required. This is used to assess the position and stability of the THR, assess for fractures and dislocation. Regular, yearly radiographs are taken to assess for THR loosening and failure.

CT scans may be required for conditions where the bony anatomy is abnormal and the surgeon wants more information such as acetabular dysplasia and following trauma. MRI scans may be used to diagnose the early stages of AVN and stage malignant tumours but provide little information for surgical planning of THR.

Post-operative management

Medical management

Patients are normally admitted on the day of surgery. The operation is performed under general or regional (spinal or epidural) anaesthesia and takes between 1 and 3 hours. In some patients an epidural catheter is left in situ for 48 hours to provide post-operative pain relief. The use of epidural pain relief should not prevent patients mobilizing after surgery; however, muscle power should be tested prior to standing patients.

Intravenous antibiotics are given at the start of the procedure and continued for three doses post-operatively in most cases and longer after revision hip replacement. A wound drain is commonly inserted at surgery and removed after 24 to 48 hours. The presence of a drain does not prevent the patient from mobilizing although the drainage bag should be emptied and the drain tube well secured.

Most patients will require a blood transfusion during or after surgery. Post-operative anaemia and postural hypotension are the main medical problems that restrict mobility. Post-operative pain can usually be controlled to allow early mobilization.

Physiotherapy management

Patients may be nursed in bed with a Charnley (abduction) pillow (Fig. 6.4). If a Charnley pillow is not available then the patient should be instructed to lie with their legs abducted (Fig. 6.5). There is often a wound drain in situ and the patient may be utilizing pain relief. Pain relief may be in the form of oral medication or most commonly as PCA (patient-controlled analgesia). PCA allows the patient to administer their own pain relief when they choose. It is worth asking the patient to prepare for physiotherapy by ensuring that their pain is covered adequately by medication prior to the commencement of treatment.

Whilst flexion less than 90° is not a specific contraindication, care should be taken whilst attempting to sit the patient forward in bed as the patient may lack flexion due to pain or post-operative stiffness. Post-operative exercises on day 1 that can be instigated include:

- Deep breath and coughing exercises.
- Foot and ankle exercises.
- Static and inner range quads.
- Active assisted hip and knee flexion.
- Active assisted hip abduction.
- Static gluteal contractions.

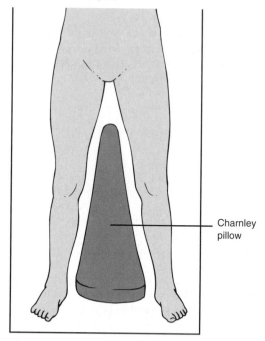

Charnley
pillow

Figure 6.4. Charnley (abduction)
pillow.

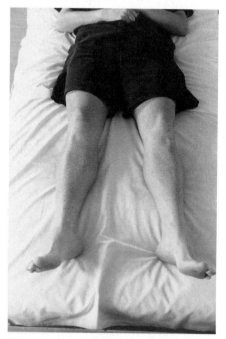

Figure 6.5. Patients should lie in
abduction if a Charnley pillow is not
available.

Mobilization can usually be commenced on day 1 or 2 post-operatively depending on the patient's physical and medical status, e.g. alertness, haemoglobin levels, blood pressure. If for any reason the patient is unable to be mobilized, then the aim should be to at least sit the patient out of bed on day 1.

The patient should generally be able to FWB or WBAT but the surgeon will advise on how much weight can be taken through the affected leg. Two physiotherapists will be needed on the first attempt to stand, with due care and consideration for nausea and dizziness. It may be necessary to commence with a frame for the first few days until balance, stability and confidence are achieved. Patients may then progress to crutches if able and confident. Adequate preparation is an important factor when first getting the patient out of bed and standing. Vital signs and recent blood tests should all be checked in the patient's case notes. Particular care should be taken that the hip does not get forced into too much flexion and adduction, especially following a posterior approach where the risk of dislocation is increased. Two physiotherapists should assist the patient.

Method for standing patient out of bed following a hip replacement:

- The bed should be raised to an appropriate height so that the patient can perch on the edge without allowing much hip flexion.
- Move the patient to the side of the bed of their non-operated leg. This can be achieved by bridging and use of an overhead bar.
- Assist the patient to drop the non-operated leg over the side of the bed whilst one therapist supports the operated leg (Fig. 6.6a).
- The other therapist comes in close and 'hugs' the patient, making sure that they keep their spine as straight as possible (Fig. 6.6b).
- The patient is instructed to tuck their chin on to their chest.
- The therapists controlling the operated leg should be in charge of the lift as they are able to control the speed of the lift whilst watching the position of the operated leg.
- The patient is then slowly rotated from the lying to the perched sitting position (Fig. 6.6c–e).
- One therapist must be watching for signs of dizziness whilst the other maintains the leg position. Once the patient is stable, the frame should then be placed in position at the front of the patient.

Following THR most patients can be mobilized with full weight bearing on the first day after surgery. There was a custom of restricting weight bearing following cementless THR for 6 weeks; however, this is no longer standard practice. Patients should not be treated with prolonged bed rest due to the complications associated with immobility. Furthermore the hip joint is still loaded during bed rest and the values may exceed that during normal gait with a cane or crutches. Weight bearing may be restricted to non-weight bearing or partial weight bearing if a fracture around the THR has occurred during prosthesis insertion or after the use of bone grafts or other complex reconstruction in revision THR. Specific instructions regarding the weight-bearing status for each patient should be determined from the surgeon's post-

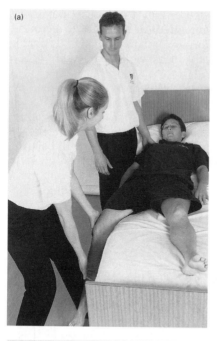

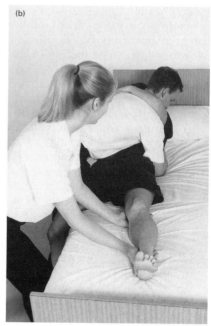

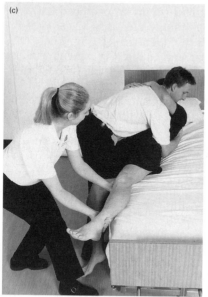

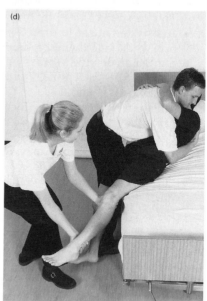

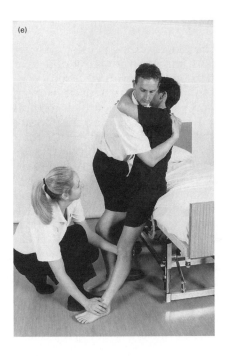

Figure 6.6. (a–e) Transferring a patient with a THR from supine lying to standing.

operative instructions which are usually noted in the operative summary. This is usually found in the patient's case notes.

The physiotherapists should continue and progress all exercises, e.g. patient may be able to achieve hip abduction in standing once able to stand. Mobilization should be progressively increased. The distance mobilized can be increased until the patient is safe and independent. Gait training should be monitored so that the patient, by discharge, develops a good, equal stride length tolerating as much weight as they are permitted. Prior to discharge it may also be necessary to instruct the patient how to manage stairs with assistive devices, depending on their home situation. Patients may also need to be taught safe transferring techniques including getting in and out of bed and sitting to stand.

At the last consultation the patient should be given advice about care of the hip at home and continuing his exercise programme. The patient should be advised to avoid sitting in low chairs; to avoid forcing the hip joint into pain and to avoid driving for the first 2–3 weeks. Patients with a posterior approach should avoid crossing their legs in sitting or lying and bending forward to put on shoes/socks or to cut their toenails. Assistive devices can be given to patients to help them with these activities.

With the current economic climate, patients are usually discharged between 5 and 7 days following the operation. Most patients do not require post-operative physiotherapy once they have been discharged. However, in many health districts there is a push for early discharge with nursing and rehabilitation to be continued in the patient's home.

Complications

Complications following THR are uncommon, occurring in less than 5 per cent of all primary THR. However, it is important to detect and treat complications early if they occur. Patients with pre-existing medical conditions and those older than 80 years are at a higher risk of developing complications and should be assessed pre-operatively and their medical condition optimized prior to surgery. Education regarding respiratory function, post-operative exercises and early mobilization will reduce complications due to bed rest and immobility. Post-operative confusion occurs in about 25 per cent of patients and results in a higher rate of complications due to falls, dislocations and wound problems.

Intra-operative complications that may delay normal mobilization include femoral or acetabular fracture, neurovascular injury and leg length inequality. Early local complications include haematoma formation, abnormal wound healing, superficial and deep wound infection, dislocation, pressure sores, deep vein thrombosis, pulmonary embolism, urinary retention and infection and general medical complications. Delayed and late complications include implant migration, breakage and loosening, heterotopic bone formation, dislocation and infection.

Dislocation

The incidence of dislocation following THR has been reported to be between 1 and 10 per cent (Morrey, 1992). Factors that contribute to an increased risk of dislocation include female gender, THR performed due to femoral neck fracture, revision THR, exposure with the posterior surgical approach, incorrect orientation of the components, alcohol intake, neurological conditions, poor muscle control and poor compliance with patients placing the hip in abnormal positions.

Sudden pain and deformity diagnose dislocation. This most commonly occurs after the patient moves to get out of bed or a chair. Plain radiography will confirm the dislocation and is used to assess for associated fractures, component malposition and loosening. The hip may dislocate posteriorly when the patient rises from sitting in a low chair, leaning forward with the legs in a position of flexion, adduction and internal rotation. Patients should be advised to sit in a high chair that does not flex the hips greater than 90° and when they stand, to do so with the feet apart and pointing forwards. Patients should avoid activities that involve bending at the hips and internal rotation. The hip may dislocate anteriorly with activities such as crossing the leg over the other when putting on socks or shoes. Aids are available to assist these activities.

The treatment involves closed reduction performed under sedation or general anaesthesia in the majority of patients. Open reduction and revision of the THR may be required in selected patients. Identification of the reason for dislocation is essential for effective treatment. Education, muscle strengthening and leg control exercises are essential in all cases and in particular for patients with poor compliance or muscle weakness.

Resting patients in bed further weakens muscle strength and leg control and is not recommended. Surgical treatment with revision THR is recommended for recurrent dislocation where component position and abductor muscle tension is abnormal.

Sciatic nerve damage

The sciatic nerve exits the pelvis through the greater sciatic notch and passes over the posterior acetabulum between the deep external rotator muscles. At the level of the hip joint, the sciatic nerve consists of two peripheral nerves: the common peroneal and tibial nerves. The two divisions are normally still joined at this level, although they may exit as separate nerves. The peroneal nerve lies most lateral and more superficial and is most likely to be damaged although the entire sciatic nerve may be involved.

This uncommon complication (0.5 to 2 per cent) will be evident by numbness of the foot or a foot drop due to ankle dorsiflexion weakness (Schmalzreid et al., 1991). Causes include stretching due to leg lengthening greater than 4 cm, trauma to the nerve by retractors or cement and local haematoma. The common peroneal nerve may also be injured by direct pressure as the nerve passes around the fibula head at the knee. Recovery is variable with poor recovery after stretching of the nerve and with patients with a severe dysaesthesia. Immediate treatment includes flexion of the hip and knee to reduce stretch on the sciatic nerve. Surgery may be indicated for removal of a large haematoma or if excessive lengthening has been performed. Further treatment includes prevention of contractures, mobilization with a foot drop splint and expectant recovery. Education is essential, as recovery is a long process, often between 18 and 24 months. The patient should have a complete explanation of the injury, timing and extent of recovery and the likely disability.

Leg length inequality

The aim of THR is to insert the THR in the correct anatomic position with normal soft tissue tension. In some cases this is not possible or an error of judgement has been made and a leg length inequality may be the result.

Leg length inequality must be carefully measured to determine if there is a true or apparent inequality. A true inequality exists when there is shortening of the skeleton. An apparent inequality may be present due to pelvic obliquity, hip flexion, and abduction or adduction contracture. Postural and gait abnormalities are common immediately after THR surgery and may mask or exaggerate a leg length inequality.

Leg length inequality may or may not cause a functional problem and patients should be assessed to determine the gait abnormality. Patients should not be treated purely on measuring the inequality and treatment does not always need to precisely correct the difference. In general, patients with an inequality less than 1 cm do not have a functional problem and they will compensate without the need of a shoe raise. Inequality between 1 and 5 cm may cause a gait abnormality and require shoe raise correction. Inequality greater than 5 cm is associated with severe gait disturbance due to differences in the level of the hip and knee joints and gait may remain abnormal despite correction of leg lengths.

Measurement of leg length inequality

True leg length – measured from greater trochanter to medial malleolus. This is a measure of inequality due to differences in bone length.
Apparent leg length – measured from xiphi-sternum to medial malleolus. This is a measure of inequality due to differences in bone leg (i.e. true length in equality) and that due to joint contractures and pelvic obliquity.

Fractures of the proximal femur

Definition

Sub-capital fracture	Intracapsular fracture of the neck of the femur (Fig. 6.7). The fracture is described as incomplete or complete and displaced or undisplaced using the Garden classification (Garden, 1964).
Intertrochanteric fracture	Proximal femoral fracture between the greater and lesser trochanters. The fracture is further described as stable or unstable based on the amount of comminution of the postero-medial femoral neck.

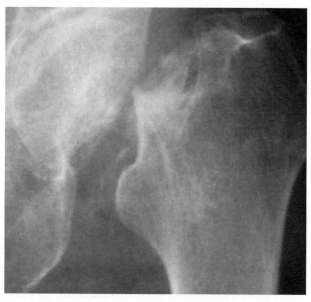

Figure 6.7. Sub-capital fracture of the neck of femur.

Hemiarthroplasty | A hip replacement where only the femoral side is replaced and therefore the artificial femoral head articulates with the normal bony acetabulum. The most common type is known as Austin–Moore prosthesis (AMP) (Fig. 6.8).

Bipolar THR | A type of hemiarthroplasty where there are two articulations between the femoral stem and the femoral head.

Fractures of the proximal femur in the elderly population are a well-documented public health problem particularly in terms of mortality, disability and cost. It has been estimated that 17–19 per cent of beds, in an orthopaedic ward, are occupied by patients with femoral neck fractures (Fenton-Lewis, 1981; Jensen et al., 1980). As life expectancy, in most Western countries, continues to increase, patients with hip fractures can be expected to place a high demand on hospital beds and resources.

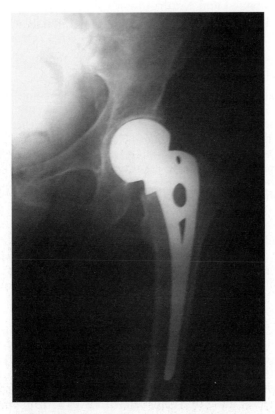

Figure 6.8. Radiograph of a hemiarthroplasty (Austin–Moore prosthesis) in situ.

Aetiology

The majority of proximal femoral fractures occur in the elderly after low velocity falls; however, the injury pattern does occur in younger patients associated with high velocity injuries (Kyle, 1994). In the elderly, the aetiology of proximal femoral fractures is multifactorial. The main factors are osteoporosis, poor balance, impaired vision and dementia. Prevention of falls by home environment modification is the most important way to reduce the incidence of proximal femoral fractures (Greenspan et al., 1994).

Incidence

Population studies on the incidence of hip fractures have been reported for several different countries (Cox et al., 1993; Hollingworth et al., 1995; Jaglal et al., 1996; Kannus et al., 1996; Nydegger et al., 1991). In the majority of these studies, the incidence of hip fractures rises exponentially after the age of 55 years. Studies have demonstrated large differences depending on geographical location, race, age and gender distribution of the population. Highest incidences have been described for Northern Europe (Scandinavia) and North America. The life-time risk for hip fracture has been reported to be between 16 to 18 per cent for women and 5 to 6 per cent for men.

Hospital requirements

Patients are assessed in the emergency department and initial medical management is commenced. This elderly group of patients often have co-existing medical problems which require acute treatment and take priority over their orthopaedic injury. Common conditions include dehydration, hypoxia and hypothermia especially if the patient has fallen in their home and not been found for several hours or days. Acute cardiac and neurological conditions may have resulted in a fall and may need assessment and treatment prior to surgery. Further delay in the orthopaedic management after initial stabilization of the patient may increase morbidity.

Coordinated care with an orthopaedic surgeon, geriatrician, physiotherapist, occupational therapist and nursing staff may improve patient function; however, there is no conclusive evidence that this management reduces morbidity, carer burden and community costs (Cameron et al., 1998).

Radiology

Antero-posterior pelvis and lateral hip radiographs are performed to diagnose the fracture and plan treatment. A nuclear bone scan or MRI may be performed if a fracture is not visible but there is a high clinical suspicion. A chest radiograph is performed for all patients pre-operatively to investigate the cardiorespiratory system and assess for rib fractures and chest trauma in high velocity injuries. Common associated injuries in the elderly include fractures of the distal radius, proximal humerus and closed head injury. Fifty per cent of patients sustaining femoral fractures due to high velocity trauma have other serious injuries (Swiontkowski et al., 1984).

Surgical anatomy and treatment

The main blood supply to the femoral head is from the retinacular blood vessels that ascend in the hip capsule. Further supply is from the metaphyseal vessels and the artery of the ligamentum teres. Intracapsular fractures of the proximal femur may disrupt the blood supply to the femoral head and result in avascular necrosis and non-union. The vessels are not always disrupted and may be in spasm or be kinked (Claffey, 1960). In young patients early reduction and stabilization of the fracture may restore blood flow and reduce the incidence of avascular necrosis. Treatment is determined by the site and displacement of the fracture and therefore the likelihood of avascular necrosis and non-union, together with the age of the patient. Displaced sub-capital fractures are associated with a higher incidence of avascular necrosis and non-union compared to undisplaced fractures (Garden, 1964). Internal fixation should be attempted in all young patients. In the elderly, prosthetic replacement, with a THR or hemiarthroplasty (AMP) is the preferred option. This prevents the need for a second operation, should the fixation fail.

For intertrochanteric fractures, the proximal femur can be separated into four parts for descriptive purposes, namely the femoral head, femoral shaft and the greater and lesser trochanters. Fractures may be described as two, three or four parts depending on the number of displaced fragments.

Operative treatment is required and the principles include an anatomic reduction by closed or open methods, solid fixation with a compression hip screw (Fig. 6.9) or intramedullary device such as a hemiarthroplasty, early mobilization and prevention of complications. It is often difficult to determine the mechanical stability of the fracture fixation due to the combined effects of osteoporosis, fracture comminution and assessment of the rigidity of the fixation device. Reduced stability may be seen with severely osteoporotic bone, non-anatomic reduction, significant postero-medial comminution and surgical error with less than perfect positioning of the fixation device in the proximal femur. The weight-bearing status may have to be modified if the fracture is thought to be unstable and therefore unable to withstand the loads through the hip joint or if the patient compliance of limited weight bearing is poor. There have been recent reports that suggest restricted weight bearing is not required in compliant patients as they will limit the loading of the hip and will progressively increase the weight bearing as the fracture heals (Koval et al., 1998).

Physiotherapy management

Physiotherapy management for patients who have had ORIF or a hemiarthroplasty follows a similar protocol to THR. However there are usually

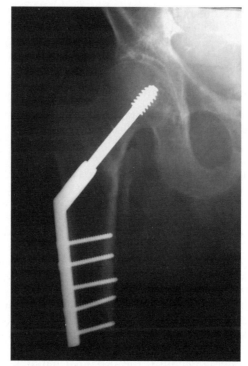

Figure 6.9. Radiograph of a compression hip screw in situ.

no precautions or contraindications and the patient can be managed with similar exercises and mobilization. It must be remembered however that these patients have undergone trauma and are usually frightened, confused and anxious. Time must be spent with the patient providing reassurance and education.

Complications

General medical problems

Early mobilization is recommended to reduce complications following fractures of the proximal femur. Post-operative anaemia, pressure sores, chest problems (atelectasis, pneumonia, pulmonary oedema), venous thrombosis and urinary retention and infection are all problems likely to affect the elderly age group. It may be necessary to restrict mobility if there is concern of myocardial infarction or ischaemia, anaemia resulting in postural hypotension or in patients who have a proximal venous thrombosis or pulmonary embolus who are not fully anti-coagulated.

Patients with post-operative confusion or poor compliance require close supervision with mobilization to prevent further falls or excessive loading of the proximal femur.

AVN and non-union and implant failure

These complications will not be evident during the hospital stay following the fracture and will not delay immediate mobilization. They will present with pain and reduction in mobility between 3 and 12 months after the fracture. Avascular necrosis and non-union can be assessed with plain radiographs and MRI in selected cases. The treatment may involve femoral osteotomy or THR in symptomatic patients in otherwise healthy and functional patients.

Implant failure may occur if the fracture fails to unite or if the bone is severely osteoporotic resulting in the screws cutting out of the femoral head. Treatment is with THR.

Hip arthroscopy

Hip arthroscopy is an evolving technique and the indications have not yet been completely defined. The main indications are for the treatment of mechanical hip pain due to acetabular tears following trauma, removal of loose and foreign bodies, assessment and treatment of articular cartilage defects and for synovial biopsy. It may have a role in staging osteonecrosis of the femoral head and early OA if non-arthroplasty treatment is being considered. Hip arthroscopy has been used to accurately assess the early stages of hip OA and determine prognosis (McCarthy and Busconi, 1995; Santori and Villar, 1999). There is no literature to suggest that procedures performed during hip arthroscopy alter the natural history of osteoarthritis.

The most common location for labral tears is the anterior sector with radial flap tears being the most common type (Farjo et al., 1999; Lage et al., 1996). Patients with labral tears and normal articular cartilage have a better prognosis compared to patients with radiographic evidence of OA and arthroscopic evidence of chondromalacia (Farjo et al., 1999).

Hip arthroscopy can be performed in the lateral or supine position. Distraction of the hip joint is obtained by significant longitudinal distraction and fluid distension. Usually two portals are created superior to the greater trochanter: one for the scope and the other for the introduction of mechanical or electrothermal instruments. The main potential complications are neuropraxia secondary to distraction and direct pressure, infection, haematoma and wound healing problems.

Patients are treated as day surgery or may require an overnight stay. There are no specific restrictions on post-operative mobility. Patients can be mobilized as tolerated with pain as a guide. Most patients are young and will not require assistive mobility devices. As most labral tears are located in the anterior sector, restriction of flexion, internal rotation and adduction may assist with pain relief.

Post-operative hip exercises

Following hip surgery the most important muscles to rehabilitate are the hip abductors and extensors as well as the knee extensors.

Static gluteal contractions

Position: Supine lying.
Instruction: Firmly squeeze your buttocks together. Hold the squeeze for 5 seconds. Relax for 5 seconds.

Active assisted or active hip flexion

Position: Supine lying.
Instruction: Bend your knee and slide on the bed towards your buttock.

The physiotherapist can assist this action if the patient is in significant pain post-operatively. It is also important, following a THR, that the patient is reminded not to let the knee drop into internal rotation as they perform this exercise.

Active or active-assisted hip abduction (Fig. 6.10)

Position: Supine lying.
Instruction: Keeping your knee straight, slowly slide your leg out away from your body.

A sliding board or assistance from the physiotherapist may be required to achieve hip abduction in the early post-operative period.

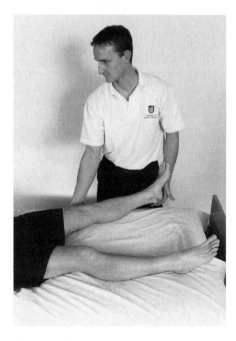

Figure 6.10. Active-assisted hip abduction.

Inner range and static quadriceps exercises

These are outlined in Chapter 6 and should be performed after hip surgery. Straight leg raise should not be given after a hemiarthroplasty or THR due to unnecessary force being applied to the new hip joint.

Bridging (Fig. 6.11)

Position: Crook-lying.
Instruction: Keep your knees and feet in line with your shoulders and your feet flat on the bed. Bend your knees to a right angle whilst pointing your knees at the ceiling. Raise your buttocks off the bed to be in line with your knees. Hold for 5 seconds and then slowly lower your buttocks to the bed.

Once patients are safe in standing, exercises should be progressed where possible:

Hip abduction and extension

Position: Standing at parallel bars or similar support.
Instruction: Keeping your knee straight, lift your leg directly out to the side and then bring it slowly back to the midline. The leg can be lifted back for hip extension. Make sure that the patient does not extend the lumbar spine.

It is important following a THR that patients keep their toes and knee pointing outwards during abduction, thereby avoiding internal rotation of the hip.

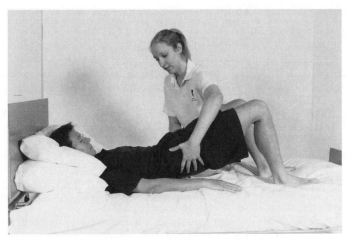

Figure 6.11. Bridging.

References

Bourne, R. B. and Kim, P. R. (1998). Cost effectiveness of total hip arthroplasty. In *The Adult Hip* (J. J. Callaghan, A G. Rosenberg and H. E. Rubash, eds.) pp. 839, Lippincott-Raven.

Butler, G. S., Hurley, C. A., Buchanen, K. L. and Smith-Van Horne, J. (1996). Prehospital education: effectiveness with total hip replacement surgery patients. *Patient Educ. Couns*, **29**, 189–197.

Cameron, I., Finnegan, T., Madhok, R., Langhorne, P. et al. (1998). Effectiveness of co-ordinated multidisciplinary inpatient rehabilitation for elderly patients with proximal femoral fracture (Cochrane Review). In *The Cochrane Library*, Issue 4, 1998.

Campbell, D. G., Masri, B. A., Garbuz, D. S. and Duncan C. P. (1998). Seven specialized exposures for revision hip and knee replacement. *Orthop. Clin. North Am.*, **29**, 229–240.

Claffey, T. J. (1960). Avascular necrosis of the femoral head. An anatomical study. *J. Bone Joint Surg.*, **42B**, 802–809.

Cox, M. A., Bowie, R. and Horne, G. (1993). Hip fractures: an increasing health care cost. *J. Orthopaed. Trauma*, **7**, 52–57.

Farjo, L. A., Glick, J. M. and Sampson, T. G. (1999). Hip arthroscopy for acetabular labral tears. *Arthroscopy*, **15**, 132–137.

Franzen, H., Johnsson, R. and Nillsson, L. T. (1997). Impaired quality of life 10 to 20 years after primary hip replacement. *J. Arthroplasty*, **12**, 21–24.

Fender, D., Harper, W. M. and Gregg, P. J. (1999). Outcome of Charnley total hip replacement across a single health region in England. *J. Bone Joint Surg.*, **81B**, 577–581.

Fenton-Lewis, A. (1981). Fracture of the neck of femur: changing incidence. *BMJ*, **283**, 1217–1220.

Garden, R. S. (1964). Stability and union in subcapital fractures of the femur. *J. Bone Joint Surg.*, **46B**, 630–647.

Gogia, P. P., Christensen, C. M. and Schmidt, C. (1994). Total hip replacement in patients with osteoarthritis of the hip: improvement in pain and functional status. *Orthopedics*, **17**, 145–150.

Greenspan, S. L., Myers, E. R., Maitland L. A, Resnick, N. M. et al. (1994). Fall severity and bone mineral density as risk factors for hip fractures in ambulatory elderly. *J. Am. Med. Assoc.*, **271**, 128–133.

Hollingworth, W., Todd, C. J. and Parker, M. J. (1995). The cost of treating hip fractures in the twenty-first century. *J. Public Health Med.*, **17**, 269–276.

Jaglal, S. B., Sherry, P. G. and Schatzker, J. (1996). The impact and consequence of hip fracture in Ontario. *Can. J. Surg.* **39**, 105–111.

Jensen, J. S., Tondevold, E. and Sorensen, P. H. (1980). Costs of treatment of hip fracture. *Acta Orthop. Scand.*, **51**, 289–296.

Kannus, P., Parkkari, J., Sievanen, H., Hienonen, A. et al. (1996). Epidemiology of fractures. *Bone*, **18**, 57S–63S.

Koval, K. J., Sala, D. A., Kummer, F. J. and Zuckerman, J. D. (1998). Postoperative weight-bearing after a fracture of the femoral neck or an intertrochanteric fracture. *J. Bone Joint Surg.*, **80A**, 352–364.

Kyle, R. F. (1994). Fractures of the proximal femur. *J. Bone Joint Surg.*, **76A**, 924–950.

Lage, L. A., Patel, J. V. and Villar, R. N. (1996). The acetabular labral tear: an arthroscopic classification. *Arthroscopy*, **12**, 269–272.

Malchau, H. and Herberts, P. (1998). Prognosis of total hip replacement. Revision and re-revision rate in THR. A revision-risk study of 148,359 primary operations. AAOS 65th Annual Meeting, Scientific Exhibit. (http://www.jru.orthop.gu.se).

McCarthy, J. C. and Busconi, B. (1995). The role of hip arthroscopy in the diagnosis and treatment of hip disease. *Can. J. Surg.*, **38** (Suppl. 1), S13–17.

Morrey, B. F. (1992). Instability after total hip arthroplasty. *Orthop. Clin. North Am.*, **23** (2), 237–247.

Muirhead-Allwood, S. K. (1998). Lessons of a hip failure. *BMJ*, **316**, 644.

NHS Centre for Reviews and Dissemination (1996). Total hip replacement – effective health care. *NHS Centre for Reviews and Dissemination*, **2**, 1–12.

Nydegger, V., Rizzoli, R., Rapin, C. H., Vasey, H. et al. (1991). Epidemiology of fractures of the proximal femur in Geneva: incidence, clinical and social aspects. *Osteoporosis Int.*, **2**, 42–47.

O'Boyle, C. A., McGee, H., Hickey, A., O'Malley, K. et al. (1992). Individual quality of life in patients undergoing hip replacement. *Lancet,* **339**, 1088–1091.

Rissanen, P., Aro, H., Sintonen, P. et al. (1996). Quality of life and functional ability in hip and knee replacements: a prospective study. *Quality of Life Res.*, **5**, 56–64.

Robinson, A. H. N., Palmer, C. R. and Villar, R. N. (1999). Is revision as good as primary hip replacement. *J. Bone Joint Surg.*, **81B**, 42–45.

Rorebeck, C. H., Bourne, R. B., Laupacis, A. et al. (1994). A double blind study of 250 cases comparing cemented with cementless total hip arthroplasty cost effectiveness and its impact on health related quality of life. *Clin. Orthop.*, **298**, 156–164.

Santori, N. and Villar, R. N. (1999). Arthroscopic findings in the initial stage of hip osteoarthritis. *Orthopaedics*, **22** (4), 405–409.

Schmalzreid, T. P., Amstutz, H. C. and Dorrey, F. J. (1991). Nerve palsy associated with total hip replacement. *J. Bone Joint Surg.* **73A**, 1074–1080.

Swedish Hip Registry. http://www.jru.orthop.gu.se

Swiontkowski, M. F., Winquist, R. A. and Hansen, S. T. Jr. (1984). Fractures of the femoral neck in patients between the ages of twelve and forty-nine years. *J. Bone Joint Surg.*, **66A**, 837–846.

Wroblewski, B. M. and Siney, P. D. (1993). Charnley low friction arthroplasty of the hip – long term results. *Clin. Orthop.*, **292**: 191–201.

CHAPTER 7

Knee surgery

The knee is an extremely complex anatomical region consisting of muscle, ligament, bone, tendon and other tissue. Surgery to the knee varies from simple procedures, such as arthroscopic evaluation, to the more complex ligamentous reconstruction and joint replacement. Physiotherapists need to have a detailed understanding of, not only the anatomy and biomechanics of the knee, but the surgical procedures, so that effective post-operative rehabilitation can be performed. General principles governing any post-operative rehabilitation include strengthening the surrounding musculature. The quadriceps (particularly vastus medialis) and the hamstrings must be strengthened to ensure successful outcome. An outline of the exercises will be given at the end of this chapter.

Total knee replacement

Total knee replacement (TKR) is a very successful operation with 90 to 95 per cent survivorship (not requiring revision) at 10 to 15 years for some designs (Martin et al., 1998; Ranawat et al., 1994; Schai et al., 1998). Several unresolved controversies remain that influence the type and technique of surgery performed. Firstly, the issue of whether to retain, sacrifice or substitute the posterior cruciate ligament (PCL). However, the 10 year results are similar for each design (Martin et al., 1998). Secondly, there is much debate around the difference between cement or cementless implants. However, the use of cement for securing the femoral and tibial implants remains the gold standard. Finally, conflict exists around whether to resurface the patella or not. These issues, on the whole, do not influence either the post-operative management of the patient or the early clinical results.

Definitions

Knee joint

The knee joint is a type of hinge joint with complex kinematics and biomechanics consisting of three articulations: the medial and lateral tibiofemoral joints and the patellofemoral articulation.

Total knee replacement

The femoral and tibial joint surfaces are re-surfaced with metal components and a polyethylene insert fits in between (Fig. 7.1). The patella is not always resurfaced. The implants may be cemented or cementless depending on the surgeon's choice.

Unicompartmental knee replacement

This procedure is indicated for painful arthrosis of either the medial or lateral compartment of the knee where only one compartment is resurfaced, commonly the medial. This procedure requires minimal disease in the other two compartments and a stable knee that has intact anterior cruciate ligament (ACL) and collateral ligaments with minor deformity. Therefore, it is not a suitable option for many patients and in most centres this operation accounts for 10 per cent of all knee replacements. In this procedure the patella is not dislocated and the quadriceps mechanism is not cut. This allows for a faster post-operative rehabilitation programme.

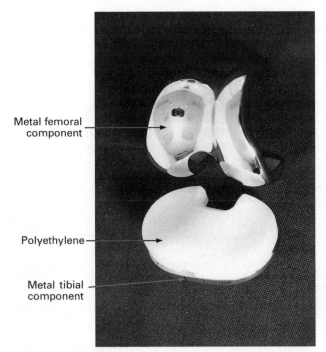

Metal femoral component

Polyethylene

Metal tibial component

Figure 7.1. Metal femoral component and polyethylene tibial component.

Indications for TKR

- Osteoarthritis of the knee can be primary or secondary and can involve either or both of the medial and lateral compartments as well as the patellofemoral articulation (Fig. 7.2). Previous partial or total menisectomy predisposes patients to osteoarthritis.
- Rheumatoid arthritis (RA).
- Post-traumatic arthritis following intra-articular fractures of the tibial plateau and distal femur.
- Avascular necrosis. This is most commonly seen in middle age women with an acute arthrosis and radiographic changes affecting the medial femoral condyle.

Hospital requirements

The hospital requirements are similar to THR although patients may often require a shorter length of stay. In the USA, patients are discharged day 3 to 4 after surgery and have home nursing and physiotherapy visits. In Australia, the average length of stay in hospital is between 7 and 10 days.

There can be difficulties in mobilizing patients that have severe bilateral fixed flexion or varus deformities and have had only one side corrected with TKR. These patients are uncommon. However, patients with severe bilateral symptoms should be considered for bilateral TKR if medically suitable. Bilateral TKR has significantly higher complication rates which makes this option unsuitable for the majority of patients with mild bilateral OA. These patients are best treated with staged procedures 3–6 months apart.

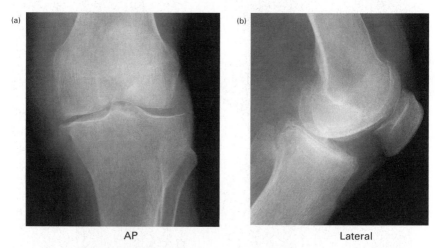

(a)   (b)

AP   Lateral

Figure 7.2. (a, b) A-P and lateral radiograph of right knee showing OA of the medial joint compartment (notice the loss of joint space on the medial side compared to the lateral).

Radiology

Standing radiographs include an A-P, lateral and skyline view (Fig. 7.3). The skyline view allows assessment of the patellofemoral joint. The radiographs are used to diagnose pathology affecting the knee joint and to plan the surgical procedure. Some surgeons use long leg, hip–knee–ankle radiographs to assess the anatomic and mechanical axes prior to surgery. Plastic templates are used to determine the correct size of implants that will restore the anatomy of the knee joint.

Post-operatively the TKR is assessed with plain radiography and an A-P and lateral view are required. This is used to assess the position of the implants and to exclude fractures. Following this, regular, yearly radiographs are taken to assess for TKR loosening and failure.

Surgical anatomy and treatment

Total knee replacement is performed under general or regional anaesthetic and usually takes between 60 to 90 minutes for primary surgery and up to 3 to 4 hours for revision surgery. A lower limb tourniquet is usually used unless there is a history of peripheral vascular disease.

A midline longitudinal skin incision is made and the knee joint is opened by incising along the medial border of the patella and patellar tendon. This is called a medial parapatellar approach. The patella can then be everted and the knee joint exposed to perform the operation. This approach may divide the infrapatellar branch of the saphenous nerve and result in numbness over the anterior proximal tibia. The extensor

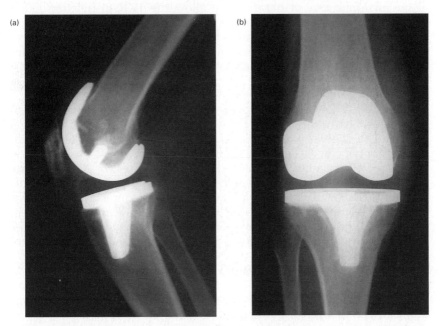

(a) (b)

Figure 7.3. (a, b) A-P and lateral view of a total knee replacement in situ.

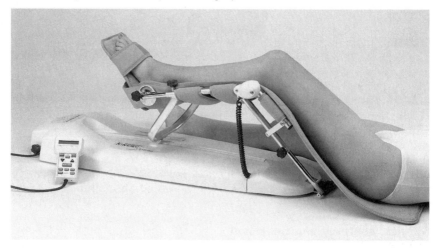

Figure 7.4. A CPM machine with a patient control attachment (reproduced with permission from Smith and Nephew).

mechanism is temporarily weakened after TKR due to the surgical incision, haematoma in and around the knee joint and altered knee joint mechanics.

Special jigs are used to cut the bone ends in the correct anatomical position and allow the implantation of the TKR. The femoral implant is placed in 5 to 7° of anatomic valgus and the tibia is placed perpendicular to the anatomic axis of the tibia. To allow the TKR to function like a normal knee, the collateral ligaments must be stable throughout the entire range of motion. An essential part of the surgery is to ensure that ligament contractures are released and that the bone cuts result in an equal space with the knee in flexion and extension. This ensures that the knee is stable and that flexion and extension are not restricted. The range of motion should be 0 to 120° at the time of surgery.

Release of all contracted ligaments and correct bone cuts should ensure that the patella moves in the groove of the femoral implant. A lateral release of the lateral parapatellar soft tissues may be required in 10–20 per cent of patients to enable normal patella tracking.

The medial incision is then sutured and a drain inserted. Antibiotics are given during surgery and for 24 hours until the drain is removed. Patients are allowed to mobilize the day after surgery. Most surgeons allow weight bearing as tolerated. Splints are not routinely used. Restriction of weight bearing and the application of a splint may be indicated after some revision TKR procedures, where bone grafts have been used, and if a fracture occurs around the implants.

Some surgeons use continuous passive motion (CPM) devices to encourage motion after surgery (Fig. 7.4). Studies have shown that CPM compared to normal mobilization may be responsible for increased blood drainage and analgesia requirement. In addition no difference in range of motion has been found 1 year after surgery (Pope et al., 1997). CPM may be useful to encourage early ROM in very anxious patients and perhaps give some psychological benefit.

Post-operative management

Medical

Analgesia is usually given with an epidural or PCA for the first 48 hours and then orally. Drains are usually removed the day after surgery and antibiotics are given in the first 24 hours following surgery. Intravenous fluids and oxygen are often required for the first 24 to 48 hours and blood transfusion may be required in this period depending on the day 1 post-operative haemoglobin levels. Patients can be mobilized with 'drips and drains' in situ; however, their early removal encourages mobilization.

Physiotherapy

Like THR, patients should be seen by the physiotherapist prior to surgery. Specific exercises can be taught along with education in the use of walking aids. Any adaptations to the home environment, such as hand rails, can also be made prior to the surgery. In addition, any factors that may affect the rate of progression need to be noted. For example, a rheumatoid patient may have upper limb joints affected which may alter their ability to effectively use walking aids.

Many surgeons use ice or cryocuffs on the knee immediately post-operatively. Ice can be applied in the form of an ice pack with due consideration for infection control or via a cryocuff. Webb et al. (1998) conducted a prospective controlled study with 20 patients using cold compressive dressings and 20 using wool and crepe dressings following TKR. Patients using the cold compressive dressings were found to have less blood loss and pain than the control group.

Exercises

- Foot and ankle exercises and deep breathe and cough – Due to the age of most patients undergoing TKR and the likelihood of concomitant medical problems, attention must be paid to performing the above exercises until the patient is mobile.
- Quadriceps strengthening – The quadriceps muscle is the most important contributor to the stability and strength of the knee. Initially the patient can focus on inner range and static quadriceps, eventually progressing to straight leg raises.
- Active or active-assisted knee flexion – This can be performed in lying on the bed or once the patient can transfer with minimal support, in sitting. Active-assisted knee flexion should be attempted first, progressing to independent active movement. Most surgeons aim for patients to achieve 90° of knee flexion prior to discharge. Therefore it is important to instigate knee flexion as soon as possible post-operatively. Most patients will find this painful due to the anterior incision site and many complain that they feel like their incision

site will break open whilst flexing the knee. The importance of requiring knee flexion for activities of daily living, such as maintaining normal gait and climbing stairs, should be explained to the patient to gain compliance. Proprioceptive neuromuscular techniques in the form of hold–relax and contract–relax may be used to facilitate gains in range of knee flexion.

- Extension ROM – It is also important that the patient does not develop a flexion contracture. The patient should be instructed to rest with the knee in extension. They should not place a pillow under the knee which would maintain the joint in a resting position of flexion. Exercises and stretches to achieve full extension should be performed.
- Gait education – Patients are usually expected to sit out of bed on the first post-operative day. Two physiotherapists should supervise and instruct the patient as many patients feel nauseous and dizzy when first sitting up. A frame will assist in the transfer and a few steps may be taken. Patients can usually weight bear as tolerated. Initial weight bearing and knee flexion may be painful due to the position of the intra-articular drain and it can be useful to wait until the drains have been removed before attempting to stand. Patients should be able to walk a few steps, which can be gradually increased until independent. Once confident, and if able, they then may progress to using two sticks. Prior to discharge, it should be ascertained if the patient has stairs or steps to negotiate at home and use of the walking aids to assist with this should be taught.

Complications

Wound healing

Soft tissue care by the surgeon is most important to reduce wound problems. Patient factors such as steroid use, diabetes, obesity, malnutrition, rheumatoid arthritis, NSAIDs and chemotherapy may all contribute to wound healing problems. If a CPM is used, it should be restricted to less than 40° flexion for the first 4 post-operative days and the knee should not be left in a flexed position. Wound drainage occurring for longer than 5 days is a concern and usually requires open debridement, culture of the causative organism and antibiotic treatment.

Neurovascular

Peroneal nerve palsy is uncommon (less than 1 per cent); however, it is the most frequent nerve palsy following TKR. It may be caused by a traction injury during surgery, tight and occlusive dressings or splints. In addition to this, there is an increased risk of peroneal nerve palsy for patients with valgus deformity greater than 20° prior to surgery. If nerve palsy is found immediately after surgery, all dressings should be removed, the knee should be flexed to 30° and the patient should be managed conservatively. Complete recovery is rare.

Direct injury to the neurovascular structures at the back of the knee may occur during surgery and should be assessed post-operatively by examination of the foot pulses, sensation and motor function.

Infection

There is a 2 per cent risk of infection following TKR, most commonly with *Staphylococcus aureus* and *Staphylococcus epidermidis*. The incidence can be reduced with antibiotics at the time of surgery and continued for 24 hours. There is a further risk with open wounds on other parts of the body, previous infection, RA, steroids and previous operations on the same knee.

Stiffness

Post-operative stiffness with ROM less than 10 through to 80° is associated with pain and decreased function. This may be due to post-operative pain, flexion–extension imbalance, an oversized femoral component or patello-femoral dysfunction. Initial treatment is to mobilize the knee and this should continue for 2–3 months. Thus patients with poor ROM on discharge should be referred for ongoing out-patient physiotherapy management. Patients that have flexion less than 80° at 3 months with no change over the preceding 4 weeks should be considered for manipulation under anaesthesia (MUA). The results of MUA are variable but may result in a small increase to allow a functional range of motion (Esler et al., 1999).

Knee arthroscopy

Arthroscopy of the knee is widely performed for a variety of conditions including knee pain following sport-related injuries and arthritis. An endoscope is inserted into the joint allowing direct visualization. This is performed through a very small incision. Many open procedures are now being performed arthroscopically with the aim of reducing patient morbidity, earlier return to sport and daily activities and a reduced hospital length of stay.

Definition of techniques performed arthroscopically

Chondroplasty

This is performed for partial thickness articular cartilage defects. It involves removal of damaged articular cartilage to make the joint surface smooth.

Osteoplasty

This is performed for full thickness articular cartilage defects. It involves burring, drilling or micro-fracture of the bone below the cartilage to encourage bleeding into the defect and a fibro-cartilaginous repair of the articular cartilage defects.

Lateral release

This involves a release of the lateral patella retinaculum and is performed to assist the normal tracking of the patella in the femoral notch. It can be performed in isolation in patients with patellofemoral dysfunction or can be performed during a TKR (10–15 per cent of all TKR) to assist tracking of the patella in the femoral notch.

Menisectomy

Resection of a torn or degenerative meniscus. This may be partial, sub-total or total (Fig. 7.5).

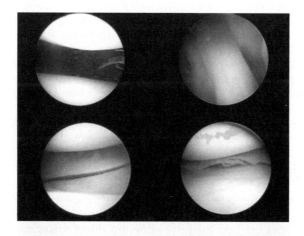

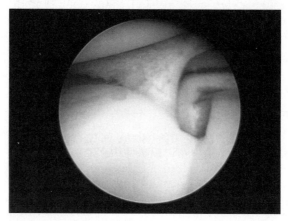

Figure 7.5. Arthroscopic visualization of the knee demonstrating a torn meniscus.

Meniscal repair

The menisci are fibrocartilage structures that have a blood supply from the peripheral peri-meniscal plexus that penetrates only the outer 25 per cent. The function is for load distribution, shock absorption, joint lubrication and as a secondary stabilizer of the knee. The peripheral blood supply can initiate a healing response only in the outer 25 per cent and therefore these tears should be repaired with meniscal sutures or resorbable suture tacks. Tears within the inner 75 per cent lack a blood supply and will not heal and are usually resected.

Hospital requirements

Most arthroscopic procedures are performed in Day Surgery Units (DSU) with patients being discharged on the same day of the surgery. Patients with complicated medical histories may be admitted overnight for observations.

Surgical anatomy and treatment

Arthroscopy of the knee is performed under general, regional or local anaesthesia. Two primary portals are made antero-medial and antero-lateral to the patella tendon at the level of the joint line to allow the arthroscope and operating instruments to be inserted into the knee joint. A third portal may be made supero-laterally for a drainage tube and several other portals may be used in special cases. First a standard inspection of the entire knee joint is carried out. Then any procedures are performed. The aim of all procedures to the meniscus or articular cartilage is to stabilize any tears and smooth the surfaces so that the knee can move freely without locking or catching on loose tissue. Small dressings (Steri-strips) are used to close the portals and a bandage is applied at the end of the arthroscopy. The bandage can be removed after 3 days.

Rehabilitation will differ depending on the procedure performed. After menisectomy and minor chondroplasty, patients can usually mobilize as tolerated and return to normal activities and sport as soon as comfort allows. After meniscal repair, range of motion is restricted to between 0–90° and weight bearing is restricted for 6 weeks. Deep squats are not allowed for 6 months and patients may return to sport at 6 months.

Radiology

Plain radiographs should be performed on all patients prior to surgery to exclude fracture, tumour and other joint pathology. Magnetic resonance imaging (MRI) is widely used to diagnose soft tissue and some bone disorders of the knee when the diagnosis is uncertain or more information will change the surgical procedure performed. MRI should not be seen as a routine investigation for all patients with knee injuries. A normal or diagnostic arthroscopy should be an uncommon procedure when a good history and examination has been performed and when MRI has been used to investigate patients with inconsistent findings on clinical examination.

Post-operative management

Medical

Patients recover in the DSU until they are awake and alert following the anaesthetic, the pain is well controlled, and have eaten. Pain relief is usually with subcutaneous morphine whilst in recovery and oral Panadeine Forte on discharge. Patients are instructed on the post-operative management including wound care and exercises. Most patients are not seen for 2 weeks after arthroscopy and therefore education is very important. To assist compliance, most surgeons have a sheet with detailed instructions that is given to the patient on discharge.

Physiotherapy

Patients undergoing an elective arthroscopy can usually be seen by the physiotherapist prior to the surgery. Where possible, specific exercises can be demonstrated and, if necessary, gait education with crutches implemented. Following arthroscopic knee surgery most patients should be able to weight bear immediately and should be discharged with advice and information about their surgery. Exercises prescription should include the following:

- Static quadriceps.
- Passive or active-assisted knee flexion progressing to active knee.
- Inner range quadriceps.
- Straight leg raise.

With specific procedures, such as meniscal repair, patients should be instructed to avoid knee flexion beyond 90°, which includes functional activities such as squatting, climbing and bench presses. Their weight-bearing status may also be limited to partial or non-weight bearing depending on the surgeon's protocol. Conversely, with a lateral release performed for patellar mal-tracking or recurrent dislocation, the physiotherapist should encourage the patient to flex the knee as far as possible, explaining that scar tissue and fibrous tissue must not be allowed to form around the site of release. A good explanation of the surgical procedure and findings is also very helpful in these situations so that the patient understands the necessity and importance of the individual exercise programme.

Complications

Knee arthroscopy is a very safe procedure and infection and neurovascular injury are very uncommon. Antibiotics are not routinely used except when prolonged procedures are performed. Portal wound problems are uncommon but require urgent assessment if they occur as synovial fistulae can occur if left untreated.

Anterior cruciate ligament reconstruction

Complete rupture of the anterior cruciate ligament is a common injury of the knee with 70 per cent caused by sport-related injuries and 50 per cent of patients having an associated meniscal tear. However not all patients with an ACL rupture will develop functional instability and progress to osteoarthritis. It is important that all patients are assessed individually as there is no single protocol applicable to all injuries. It is also important to diagnose associated injuries to the collateral ligaments and the menisci as this may determine the need for an acute arthroscopy. Non-operative management may be indicated for patients with a low demand lifestyle and are greater than 40 years.

Definition

Lachman test

This test is to assess the integrity of the ACL and is performed with the knee in approximately 20° of flexion. One hand supports the thigh, the other hand applies an anterior force to the posterior aspect of the tibia. Tibial displacement and quality of end-feel should be noted and compared to the other knee. Abnormal end-feel and/or displacement result in a positive test. Integrity of the PCL must be established prior to performing this test to prevent false-positive results.

Pivot shift test

This is a dynamic test that demonstrates anterior laxity of the knee. The test is performed by placing the knee in extension, the foot in internal rotation and the leg slightly abducted. A hand is placed on the lateral side of the leg and applies a valgus force to the leg whilst gently flexing the knee. The test is positive with reduction of the subluxed tibia at 20–30° of flexion with the lateral femoral condyle sliding forward on the tibial plateau to a reduced position.

Open chain kinetic (OCK) exercise

An exercise or movement where the distal end segment of the limb does not meet resistance, e.g. inner range quadriceps over a rolled towel.

Closed kinetic chain (CKC) exercise

An exercise or movement where the distal end segment of the limb meets resistance, e.g. quarter squat in standing.

Continuous passive motion (CPM)

This passive motion of an extremity through an externally supplied force.

Aetiology

Johnson and Warner (1993) state that the most common mechanism for ACL rupture is a contact injury with the knee in external rotation whilst enduring a valgus stress. Such a mechanism usually results in concurrent injury to the medial collateral ligament (MCL) and medial meniscus. This is commonly termed an 'unhappy triad'. Other mechanisms included forced knee hyper-extension or a direct blow with the knee in flexion as sustained in a dashboard injury. Most commonly these injuries take place in sports such as football, soccer, netball, basketball and skiing and constitute 78 per cent of all such injuries (Lutz et al., 1990).

Indications

Indications for ACL reconstructive surgery include:

- Young, competitive participants of high speed sports that involve cutting, jumping and pivoting.
- Active patients with a concomitant repairable meniscal tear or other significant collateral ligament injuries.
- Patients who experience episodes of instability during activities of daily living (Frank and Jackson, 1997; Fu and Schulte, 1996).

Hospital requirements

Patients often stay in hospital for between 2–3 days. The patient can usually be discharged when they are mobilizing safely with a range of motion from 5 to 90° and can perform a straight leg raise. Some centres in the USA are performing ACL reconstruction as day surgery although this is uncommon in Australia.

Surgical anatomy and treatment

The ACL is the primary structure that prevents the tibia from translating anteriorly providing 85 per cent of the total resistance. The femoral attachment is on the postero-medial aspect of the lateral femoral condyle. The tibial attachment is on the central non-articular portion of the tibial plateau, between the attachments of the anterior horns of the medial and lateral menisci and anterior to the PCL attachment. Some fibres of the ACL are taut throughout all positions of knee movement.

The most common reconstruction for a torn ACL is arthroscopic reconstruction with autogenous bone–patellar tendon–bone or multiple strand hamstring grafts. These are termed autogenous grafts because the replacement ACL is taken from the patient's own body. In general, primary repair (direct suturing) of the torn ACL, prosthetic replacement, allograft ACL (an ACL taken from a tissue bank) and extra-articular soft tissue reconstruction have inferior results compared to autogenous grafts. However, some excellent short-term results have been reported with all techniques.

The bone–patellar tendon–bone graft is usually harvested from the middle third (10 mm) of the patellar tendon with 15×10 mm bone plugs at each end. Hamstring grafts are harvested at the insertion on the tibia of the semitendinosus and gracilis tendons. The tendons are doubled over to give a multiple (four strand) graft. These grafts approach the strength of the normal ACL, however some graft weakening will occur after implantation.

A standard arthroscopy of the knee is performed to assess and treat pathology of the menisci and chondral surfaces. The remnant of the ACL is debrided and the intercondylar notch is cleared of soft tissue. At this point the arthroscope is removed and the graft is harvested. Either the bone–patellar tendon–bone or hamstring graft is then prepared and measured. The arthroscope is then re-inserted and special guides are used to assist in the accurate placement of the tibial and femoral tunnels. The tunnels are made and then the graft is passed through the tunnels and checked to ensure that the graft is isometric through a full range of motion and there is no impingement of the graft with the roof of the intercondylar notch. The graft is then fixed to the femur and tibia using interference screws, staples or other devices. The knee is washed out and a drain is usually inserted.

Radiology

Plain radiographs should be performed on all patients prior to surgery to exclude fracture, tumour and other joint pathology. MRI may be used to exclude other pathology within the knee if considering non-operative management. The findings from MRI rarely alter the management of a patient with a symptomatic, clinically ACL-deficient knee and therefore is not recommended for routine use.

Post-operative management

Medical

Post-operative pain relief is with PCA, subcutaneous morphine or Panadeine Forte. Application of ice and the use of CPM are commonly used; however, there is little evidence to suggest any benefit. Patients usually commence range of motion exercises immediately although some surgeons do not like the knee to be hyperextended. Splints are not routinely used and crutches are often required for several weeks.

Physiotherapy

Most patients undergoing this procedure are between 20 and 30 years of age (Dunleavy, 1993). Therefore patients can be mobilized early and there is little risk of DVT and chest infection. If there is some concern, then prophylactic physiotherapy must be performed. ACL post-operative rehabilitation protocols are wide and varied. Protocols vary between surgeons. Close communication with the consulting surgeon should be made to ensure that the rehabilitation programme is being implemented according to their requirements.

The major controversy surrounding immediate ACL rehabilitation is the strain sustained by the healing graft tissue during the various exercises performed. There is a continuing debate surrounding the value of either closed or open kinetic chain knee extension exercises. Many authors believe that OKC knee extension exercises, specifically in the last 30°, cause anterior translation of the tibia due to quadriceps contraction. This is thought to place greater strain on the graft. However, other authors believe that some strain in the early stages may in fact assist with ligament remodelling and increasing tensile strength at the attachment sites. Thus in the last decade CKC exercises have been advocated as a safer and more effective form of exercise following ACL reconstruction. Closed chain is a functional exercise mainly performed in weight-bearing positions. They are thought to be safer due to less strain on the graft site. In addition they are thought to be better for training rectus femoris and anecdotally patients are more satisfied performing these exercises. A disadvantage with these exercises is that if a patient has a very atrophied quadriceps muscle then a CKC exercise may not be sufficient to strengthen a very weakened muscle.

The frequently accepted current general consensus is that CKC exercises should be performed early during rehabilitation until sufficient graft healing has occurred (to prevent compromising the graft), after which OKC exercises may be commenced. Theoretically, however, both OKC and CKC can be modified and performed without placing excessive strain on the graft and some *light* strain may be beneficial for graft healing (Fitzgerald, 1997).

Patellar mobilization

Passive patellar mobilization prevents contracture of the patellar retinacular tissue and arthrofibrosis (Noyes et al., 1992). The patella can be mobilized in all directions as outlined in Maitland (1991). The most important directions are medial and inferior (Fig. 7.6).

Acute care physiotherapy should therefore include:

- Foot and ankle exercises.
- Deep breathe and cough exercises.
- Quadriceps exercises (either OKC or CKC depending on surgeon preference).
- Hamstring contractions.
- Ice.
- Patellar mobilization.
- Gait re-education with or without a brace and crutches.
- Proceed to stairs.

Continuous passive motion (CPM)

Some surgeons still elect to use a CPM for patients following ACL reconstruction. However, research has suggested that the CPM is of little benefit both in the long and short term following ACL reconstruction.

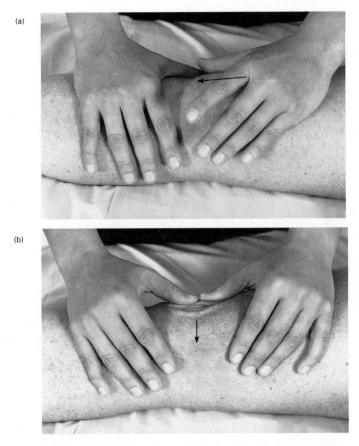

(a)

(b)

Figure 7.6. Mobilization of the patella. (a) Inferior glide.
(b) Medial glide.

Long-term rehabilitation

Traditional rehabilitation programmes following ACL reconstruction aim
to return the patient to sporting activity by 9–12 months. However, more
recently accelerated rehabilitation programmes have been developed that
seek to achieve rehabilitation milestones earlier, aiming for return to functional activities by 4–6 months. A number of studies have detailed accelerated rehabilitation programmes, and an example is included in Table
7.1. A complete review is beyond the scope of this book and the reader is
referred to a number of excellent review articles outlining the advantages
and disadvantages of these programmes (Shelbourne and Gray, 1997;
Shelbourne and Nitz, 1990; Shelbourne et al., 1995).

Complications

Arthrofibrosis is a condition where intra-articular fibrous contractures
occur that severely restrict the range of knee motion. There is a higher

Table 7.1. An example of an accelerated and traditional rehabilitation programme adapted from De Carlo et al. (1992), Shelbourne and Gray (1997), Shelbourne et al. (1995), and Shelbourne and Nitz (1990)

Time	Traditional rehabilitation protocol	Time	Accelerated rehabilitation protocol
Pre-op	• N/A	Pre-op	• ↓swelling, ↑ROM, education re: post-operative rehabilitation
1/7	• Leg splint at 45°F • Commence CPM	1/7	• ↑ROM (CPM) • Knee immobilized full E for walking • Ambulate WBAT (crutches) • ↓swelling (ice, Cryocuff)
2–3/7	• Abd, Add, SLR • PROM 0–90° • Ambulate NWB	2–4/7	• D/C (pain managed, full E, SLR, FWB)
5–6/7	• D/C • Continue exs/CPM at home • Knee immobilized (10°) walking • PWB (toe touch)	7–10/7	• ROM – full E (prone hang), active assisted flexion • Strengthening exs – knee F, step-ups, calf raises • FWB • No knee immobilizer
3/52	• Quads exs • AROM 60–90°, PROM 0–90°	2–3/52	• ROM 0–110° • Strength – single leg stance dips, calf raises • Gym – leg press, $\frac{1}{4}$ squats, bike • Swimming/hydrotherapy • Functional knee brace
6/52	• PROM 0–100 • WBAT • Functional brace	5–6/52	• ROM 0–130° • Isokinetic test (20° E block) • Jogging/agility training if strength >70% • Continue/progress gym • VMO bulk restored • Discontinue functional brace
8–10/52	• FWB/WBAT • ROM 0–110° (prone hangs if not full E) • Strength exs – resisted SLR, resisted eccentric knee E, hamstring curls, cycling • Swimming/ hydrotherapy	10/52	• Full ROM • Agility training/sports specific exs

Table 7.1. (Continued)

Time	Traditional rehabilitation protocol	Time	Accelerated rehabilitation protocol
12–14/ 52	• ROM 0–120° • FWB • Progress exs	16/52	• Agility training
4/12	• ROM 0–130° • Discontinue brace for ADLs • ↑exs intensity, weights, reps, sets, speed of isokinetics	4–6/12	• Return to full sport if full ROM, no swelling, stable knee, completed running programme
5/12	• Jumping agility exs		
6/12	• Agility exs • Distance walking		
7–8/12	• Progress strength/ agility exs • Running		
9–12/12	• Return to sport if strength >80%, full ROM, no swelling, stable knee, completed running programme		

incidence if the ACL reconstruction is performed acutely after injury or if the patient does not have a full range of motion prior to surgery. Treatment consists of range of motion exercises and in some cases arthroscopic division of adhesions and manipulation.

Re-rupture is uncommon (approximately 4 per cent) and the risk times are between 3–6 months following surgery and at the time of return to sport. In general rehabilitation exercises will only place the ACL graft under low tensile strains, well below the failure capacity of the graft. At the time of return to sport, the knee must have healing of the graft and intact secondary stabilizers to reduce the risk of re-rupture.

Complications from the donor sites have been reported. Anterior knee pain has been attributed to patella ligament graft harvesting; however, it has also been noted to be more common in patients with ACL-deficient knees treated non-operatively than in control patients. Hamstring weakness has also been reported following hamstring graft harvest; however, this is rarely symptomatic.

Knee exercises

Following any knee surgery it is vitally important to strengthen the quadriceps muscle. Pain and swelling around the knee can result in reflex inhibition of this muscle and if left untreated, will affect the long-term outcome for the patient. It is therefore imperative that quadriceps control be gained prior to discharge.

Static quadriceps exercises (Fig. 7.7)

Position: Long sitting. Therapist places one hand under the affected knee and the other hand under the patient's heel.

Instruction: 'Pull your foot and toes up towards you, then push your knee down onto my hand by tightening up the thigh muscle.'

At the same time the patient should **not** be pushing down on the hand that is under the heel. If this happens then they are performing hip rather than knee extension.

Inner range quadriceps (IRQ) (Fig. 7.8)

Position: Long sitting or supine. Place a rolled up towel under the patient's knee.

Instruction: 'Pull your foot and toes up to your nose. Then push your knee into the towel and slowly lift your heel as far as you can off the bed.'

On first attempt patients may need assistance to lift the heel. This is an OKC knee extension exercise.

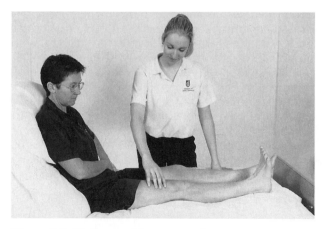

Figure 7.7. Static quadriceps exercise.

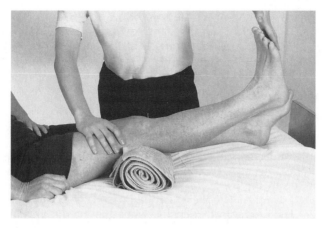

Figure 7.8. Inner range quadriceps exercise.

Straight leg raise (Fig. 7.9)

Position: Long sitting or supine lying.
Instruction: 'Pull your foot and toes up to your nose, push your knee into the bed and then slowly raise your whole leg off the bed.'

Only lift the foot approximately 10 cm off the bed. The patient should not attempt a straight leg raise until they have gained sufficient control during a static and inner range exercise. This is an OKC exercise.

Co-contraction knee exercise

If the surgeon requests that only closed kinetic chain exercises be performed, then co-contraction of the quadriceps and hamstrings can be conducted in sitting or in partial weight bearing.

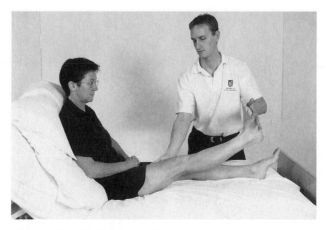

Figure 7.9. Straight leg raise.

Position: Sitting or partial weight bearing.
Instruction: 'Tighten up the hamstring muscle at the back and then the quadriceps muscle at the back of your thigh. Hold for 10 seconds and relax.'

Quadriceps lag measurement

Position: As for IRQ.
Instruction: As for IRQ.

Once the patient has extended as much as possible the therapist places one hand under the heel and supports the thigh with the other hand. Holding the leg in the extension achieved by the patient, the patient is then instructed to relax. The therapist then passively extends the knee to end of range. The amount of extension gained is the quadriceps lag.

Knee flexion in sitting or lying (Fig. 7.10)

Position: Long sitting or supine lying.
Instruction: 'Keeping your heel on the bed, slowly slide your heel up to your buttock as far as you can.'

The therapist can help by supporting the knee or instruct the patient to support the knee with their hands. This exercise can be progressed to performing knee flexion in sitting, either over the edge of the bed or in a chair.

Techniques to stimulate a muscle contraction

If there is a reflex inhibition of the quadriceps mechanism, techniques that stimulate a contraction include muscle tapping and stroking, facilitation with quick ice massage and overflow techniques (e.g. maximal contraction of the patient's other leg or arms). In cases resistant to these techniques,

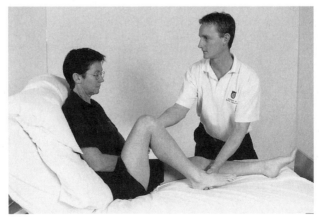

Figure 7.10. Knee flexion in lying.

electrical stimulation with either an interrupted low frequency current or bipolar interferential current may be appropriate.

References

De Carlo, M. S., Shelbourne, K. D., McCarroll, J. R. and Rettig, A. C. (1992). Traditional versus accelerated rehabilitation following ACL reconstruction: a one year follow-up. *J. Orthop. Sports Phys. Ther.*, **15**, 309–316.

Dunleavy, J. (1993). Acute care physical therapy management of arthroscopically assisted anterior cruciate ligament reconstruction. *Ortho. Phys. Ther. Clin. North Am.*, **2**, 197–205.

Esler, C. N. A., Lock, K., Harper, W. M. and Gregg, P. J. (1999). Manipulation of total knee replacements. Is the flexion gained retained? *J. Bone Joint Surg.*, **81B**, 27–29.

Fitzgerald, G. K. (1997). Open versus closed kinetic chain exercise: issues in rehabilitation after anterior cruciate ligament reconstructive surgery. *Physical Therapy*, **77**, 1747–1754.

Frank, C. B. and Jackson, D. W. (1997). The science of reconstruction of the anterior cruciate ligament. *J. Bone Joint Surg.*, **79A**, 1556–1576.

Fu, F. H. and Schulte, K. R. (1996). Anterior cruciate ligament surgery 1996 – state of the art. *Clin. Orthop.*, **325**, 19–24.

Johnson, D. L. and Warner, J. J. P. (1993). Diagnosis for anterior cruciate deficiency. *Clinics in Sports Med.*, **12**, 671–684.

Lutz, G. E., Stuart, M. J., Sim, F. H. and Scott, S. G. (1990). Rehabilitative techniques for athletes after reconstruction of the anterior cruciate ligament. *Mayo Clin. Proc.*, **65**, 1322–1355.

Maitland, G. D. (1991). *Peripheral Manipulation* pp. 221–290, Butterworth–Heinemann.

Martin, S. D., Scott, R. D. and Thornhill, T. S. (1998). Current concepts in total knee arthroplasty. *J. Orthop. Sports Phys. Ther.*, **28**, 252–261.

Noyes, F. R., Demaio, M. and Mangine, R. E. (1992). Minimal protection program: advanced weight bearing and range of motion after ACL reconstruction – weeks 1 to 5. *Orthopaedics*, **15**, 504–515.

Pope, R. O., Corcoran, S., McCaul, K. and Howie, D. W. (1997). Continuous passive motion after primary total knee replacement. Does it offer any benefits? *J. Bone Joint Surg.*, **79B**, 914–917.

Ranawat, C. S., Flynn, W. F. Jr. and Deshmukh, R. G. (1994). Impact of modern technique on long-term results of total condylar knee arthroplasty. *Clin Orthop.*, **309**, 131–135.

Schai, P. A., Thornhill, T. S. and Scott, R. D. (1998). Total knee arthroplasty with the PFC system. Results at a minimum of ten years and survivorship analysis. *J Bone Joint Surg.*, **80**, 850–858.

Shelbourne, K. D. and Gray, T. (1997). Anterior cruciate ligament reconstruction with autogenous patellar tendon graft followed by accelerated rehabilitation: a two- to nine-year followup. *Amer. J. Sports Med.*, **25**, 786–795.

Shelbourne, K. D., Klootwyk, T. E., Wilckens, J. H. and De Carlo, M. S. (1995). Ligament stability two to six years after anterior cruciate ligament reconstruction with autogenous patellar tendon graft and participation in accelerated rehabilitation program. *Amer. J Sports Med.*, **23**, 575–579.

Shelbourne, K. D. and Nitz, P. (1990). Accelerated rehabilitation after anterior cruciate ligament reconstruction. *Amer. J. Sports Med.*, **18**, 292–299.

Webb, J. M., Williams, D., Ivory, J. P., Day, S. and Williamson, D. M. (1998). The use of cold compression dressings after total knee replacement – a randomised, controlled trial. *Orthopedics*, **21**, 51–61.

CHAPTER 8

Shoulder surgery

The shoulder is the most mobile joint of the human body and allows the hand to be placed in space for prehensile activities. Movement of the shoulder joint should not be considered in isolation as the shoulder joint requires movement of the scapulo-thoracic articulation, sterno-clavicular joint and acromio-clavicular joint to obtain full elevation, abduction and rotation. Many muscle groups cross the shoulder from the body to the pectoral girdle, the pectoral girdle to the upper limb and from the body to the upper limb directly. Their role is to provide strength and stability to the shoulder.

Shoulder surgery can be performed with open procedures (arthrotomy) and with arthroscopy. Arthroscopy is used for the diagnosis of intra-articular pathology and the indications are expanding to include some procedures that were previously performed only as open procedures (Altchek, 1995; Ellman et al., 1986). The advantages of arthroscopy include lower morbidity, reduced hospital length of stay and early return to function. With experience, the results of surgery via arthroscopy are gradually improving (Lazarus et al., 1994).

The shoulder joint is prone to stiffness if not mobilized and therefore passive movement should be allowed after most shoulder operations. In general, active movement is restricted if the rotator cuff has been repaired or has been divided and repaired as part of the operation. A description of all exercises is given at the end of this chapter.

Sub-acromial decompression and rotator cuff repair

Definitions

The sub-acromial space

This is the space below the acromial arch (acromion, acromio-clavicular ligament and acromio-clavicular joint) and is separated from the shoulder joint by the sub-acromial bursa and the rotator cuff (Fig. 8.1).

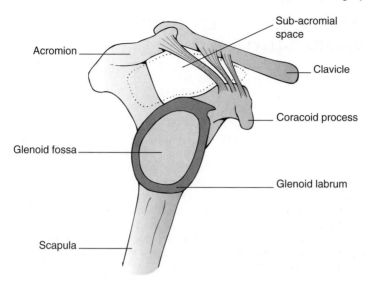

Figure 8.1. The sub-acromial space. In this space lies the sub-acromial bursa and the rotator cuff tendon.

The rotator cuff

This is a complex of four muscles (supraspinatus, infraspinatus, teres minor and subscapularis) that arise from the scapula and insert into the humerus. Their role is to assist in the stability of the shoulder, rotate the shoulder and act as a humeral head depressor during shoulder elevation and abduction.

Introduction

Matsen and Arntz (1990) define impingement as 'the encroachment of the acromion, coraco-acromial ligament, coracoid process and/or acromio-clavicular joint on the rotator cuff mechanism that passes beneath them as the glenohumeral joint is moved, particularly in flexion and rotation'. This impingement causes friction centred on the supraspinatus that may extend to the infraspinatus and the long head of biceps (LHB). This friction may eventually result in a degenerative tear of the rotator cuff tendon. Thus the impingement is a continuum ranging from inflammation or degeneration of the sub-acromial structures to partial or complete tears of the rotator cuff (Matsen and Arntz, 1990; Neer, 1972).

Neer (1972) described the pathology of impingement syndrome into three stages:

Stage I: Oedema and haemorrhage usually in young athletes involved in overhead sporting activities.

Stage II: Thickening and fibrosis with a possible rotator cuff tear.

Stage III: Tendon degeneration and complete rotator cuff tear.

Impingement syndrome and tears of the rotator cuff are common problems affecting two distinct groups of people: athletes involved with repeated overhead activity and elderly people with an increased prevalence with age greater than 70 years. Tears of the rotator cuff have a multifactorial aetiology. Many are caused by age-related degenerative changes associated with an area of reduced vascularity of the supraspinatus tendon and impingement syndrome. In addition, a number of factors may alter the normal biomechanics of the shoulder complex leading to impingement (Table 8.1). In the majority of cases, impingement syndrome is caused by a diminished space below the acromial arch and is usually associated with a hooked acromion and/or an acromial spur. In general, all acute tears should be repaired within 3 weeks, whilst symptomatic chronic tears in active, cooperative patients that have failed adequate physiotherapy and other conservative measures over a 6 month period, should be repaired (Harryman et al., 1991). The results of surgical repair are directly related to the size of the tear and the duration of pre-operative symptoms (Esch et al., 1988; Liu and Baker, 1994; Wolfgang 1974).

Table 8.1. Factors contributing to the development of impingement syndrome

Factors	Cause	
Environmental	Overuse, e.g. in paraplegics, over head athletes. Trauma, e.g. fall	
Extrinsic	Primary impingement due to:	• Outlet stenosis • AC joint degenerative joint disease with osteophyte formation • Unfused or abnormal-shaped acromion
	Secondary impingement	• Loss of normal humeral head depression mechanism or scapular rotation • Cuff tear or weakness • Minor or gross instability • Scapular muscle weakness or imbalance
Intrinsic	Tendon degeneration due to:	• Ageing • Hypovascularity of supraspinatus tendon • Bursal inflammation

Hospital requirements

Usually performed as a short stay admission. Patients are admitted on the day of surgery and discharged the day after surgery when pain is controlled and the rehabilitation programme is understood. Surgery is usually performed under general anaesthetic and therefore routine preoperative investigations such as chest X-ray (CXR), electrocardiogram (ECG) and blood tests are required for most patients over the age of 60 or with significant medical problems.

Radiology

Plain radiographs are used to assess the anatomy of the acromion and proximal humerus and to exclude other causes of shoulder pain such as glenohumeral osteoarthritis, tumours and acromio-clavicular arthritis. Ultrasound imaging is often performed to assess the rotator cuff muscles for tears and may also demonstrate impingement with dynamic imaging. Ultrasound is good for diagnosing full thickness tears with a positive predictive value of 95 per cent. If the diagnosis is negative, MRI or arthroscopy should be considered.

Surgical anatomy and treatment

The standard treatment of rotator cuff tears is an open repair of the rotator cuff and an acromioplasty. Acromioplasty involves resecting the antero-inferior surface of the acromion. Some surgeons also remove the coraco-acromial ligament to further increase the sub-acromial space. Acromioplasty is performed to remove any impingement of the rotator cuff. An acromioplasty may be performed in isolation for impingement syndrome without rotator cuff tear or in conjunction with a rotator cuff debridement or repair.

Acromioplasty can be performed by open or arthroscopic techniques. Both have demonstrated similar excellent outcomes in patients. The arthroscopic technique, whilst allowing for faster rehabilitation and early return to work, is technically demanding for the surgeon and results are often dependent on the skill and experience of the surgeon. The open procedure is a safe, reliable approach for the majority of elderly patients with a clear history of impingement syndrome and rotator cuff tears can be repaired through the same incision. The open procedure is performed through a small incision over the antero-lateral aspect of the acromion. The deltoid muscle is reflected off the acromion to expose the acromial arch. The antero-lateral acromion is resected and, as previously mentioned, the coraco-acromial ligament may be released and osteophytes removed from the acromio-clavicular joint. It is imperative that the deltoid is repaired strongly, usually with sutures passed through bone.

The advantage of the arthroscopic technique is that the intra-articular structures of the shoulder can be viewed, partial rotator cuff tears can be detected and debrided and the deltoid muscle origin is not cut to gain exposure. Therefore this technique is commonly used when there is no suspicion of an associated rotator cuff tear. The arthroscopic group have been observed to have better early range of motion and return to work; however, the results are no different at 3 months (Sachs et al., 1994).

Complications

General complications such as wound healing, haematoma and infection can occur. Adhesive capsulitis (frozen shoulder) can occur if the patient is not mobilized after surgery. As mentioned above, the results are excellent for this procedure and poor results should be assessed for other pathology or an error in the operative technique.

Deltoid muscle weakness may occur if the deltoid is not strongly re-attached to the acromion after being reflected during the open procedure or split greater than 5 cm from the acromion, resulting in damage to the axillary nerve. Persistence symptoms, after an arthroscopic acromioplasty, may be due to inadequate resection of the acromion.

Physiotherapy

To achieve the best possible outcome following any surgery to the shoulder, patients should be seen by the physiotherapist pre-operatively in a pre-admission clinic. Exercises and advice regarding the post-operative management should be given. Important subjective information to collate should include the age and general requirements of the patient, hand dominance, general fitness and expectations. In addition, strength and range of movement of the affected shoulder should be assessed and recorded.

Following any shoulder surgery pain and swelling are common complaints. Both can inhibit recovery as many patients may be unwilling to mobilize the shoulder. This could lead to the development of adhesions in the capsule resulting in a stiff tight shoulder. Small reductions in range of movement can cause significant functional deficits that can impede the patients' lifestyle (Bruzga and Speer, 1999).

Post-operative management of pain and swelling should include the use of cryocuffs or ice packs. Cryotherapy has been shown to reduce post-operative pain levels following shoulder surgery (Speer et al., 1996). In addition to ice, all physiotherapy treatments should be timed to coincide with pain relief medication to achieve the best results.

Post-operatively patients will often wear a sling. There are a variety of different devices ranging from commercially made slings that significantly confine movement to the more simple collar and cuffs or triangular bandages (Fig. 8.2). One of the most comfortable slings is the Edinburgh collar and cuff which does not result in the weight being taken through the affected shoulder but rather the contralateral side (Fig. 8.3).

Wearing of a sling may be required for comfort and for only a few days. However following reconstructive or reparative surgery the sling may be worn for as long as 6 weeks. Whilst wearing the sling, patients must be instructed in exercises to prevent muscle atrophy and joint stiffness of the rest of the upper extremity. This should include full range of elbow flexion

(a)

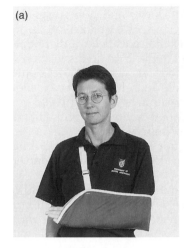

(b)

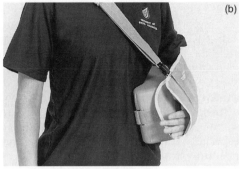

Figure 8.2. Commercially available slings.
(a) A simple supportive sling. (b) Sling
with small abduction pillow which may be
used following a rotator cuff repair.

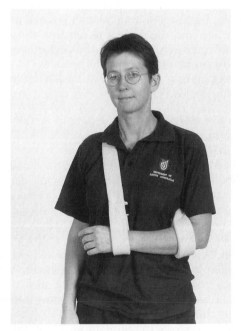

Figure 8.3. Edinburgh sling.

and extension in varying° of supination and pronation, wrist flexion and
extension as well as strengthening exercises particularly for the muscles
involved in gripping.

Strengthening exercises following shoulder surgery should concentrate
not only on the rotator cuff, which provides dynamic stability to the
joint, but also on the scapular stabilizers, which rotate the scapular
sufficiently to allow for full elevation of the shoulder (Wilk et al.,

1991). The force couple of serratus anterior, lower and upper trapezius are important for motion of the scapula and its stabilization during movement of the glenohumeral joint. Many clinicians believe that imbalance or altered recruitment of this force couple is a predisposition to glenohumeral dysfunction (Ayub, 1991; Jobe et al., 1990; McConnell, 1991). Certainly insufficient control by these muscles would not allow sufficient rotation of the scapula for overhead activities and could predispose to impingement syndrome. Therefore it is vital that strength and stability of these muscles is maintained or improved following surgery especially if the arm is confined to a sling for long periods. In addition, posture retraining and advice should also be implemented to prevent protracted and elevated scapular position.

Following an open or arthroscopic acromioplasty, patients should be instructed in exercises for achieving passive elevation and external rotation. This may be performed for impingement or in the presence of an irreparable massive rotator cuff tear. Neer (1983) found that patients with irreparable massive tears of the rotator cuff can be made more comfortable and achieve improvements in function following acromioplasty alone. In open techniques, the surgeon may restrict passive motion if the deltoid repair was not strong and the patient rested in a sling for 6 weeks. If an acromioplasty and rotator cuff repair were performed then active movement will be restricted for 4–6 weeks.

Therefore post-operative exercise prescription following sub-acromial decompression with or without rotator cuff repair should include:

- Foot and ankle exercises until the patient is mobile.
- Deep breath and cough exercises.
- Elbow and hand exercises.
- Active assisted flexion progressing to active flexion. Passive or auto-assisted flexion can be performed following a rotator cuff repair. However, active abduction should be avoided for 4–6 weeks. Patients should be advised to avoid heavy lifting and any excessive active movement for the first 6 weeks. However, passive range is important to prevent any unwanted stiffness of the shoulder. Passive exercise can be performed in the following exercises: auto-assisted flexion in lying using the contra-lateral arm to assist; pendular exercises, use of a pulley device or a stick.
- Pendular exercises in or out of sling avoiding abduction movements if the rotator cuff was repaired.
- Resisted static exercises to maintain muscle strength. Resisted static adduction, extension and internal rotation can be performed. However, following a rotator cuff repair, resisted external rotation and abduction should be avoided.
- Shoulder girdle retraction and depression. In all shoulder surgery it is very important to maintain the length and strength of the shoulder girdle muscles.
- Postural education.

Shoulder arthroplasty

Shoulder arthroplasty involves resurfacing or replacing the articulating surfaces of the humeral head and the glenoid. Compared to hip and knee joint replacements, shoulder arthroplasty is a relatively new and developing technique. New techniques, implants and indications have been advanced over the years such that the outcomes of shoulder arthroplasty are consistently improving. The main indications for shoulder arthroplasty are debilitating pain and, to a lesser extent, limitations in range of motion and strength. Indications for shoulder replacement surgery therefore include osteoarthritis, rheumatoid arthritis, post-traumatic arthritis and displaced and comminuted fractures of the humeral head. The best results are achieved in patients with preserved bone stock, an intact rotator cuff and those that have been well prepared for the extensive rehabilitation. Hence patients with osteoarthritis generally have better results than rheumatoid arthritis. Rheumatoid arthritis patients tend to have excellent improvement in pain but only a small improvement in range of movement due to rotator cuff weakness. Generally, a 10 year implant survivorship has been demonstrated in 75–90 per cent of cases (Boileau and Walch, 1997; Neer et al., 1982; Hawkins et al., 1989).

Types of shoulder arthroplasty

Total shoulder arthroplasty (TSA)

Replacement of both the humeral and glenoid surfaces of the shoulder.

Unconstrained TSA

The artificial humeral head articulates with the glenoid component. This is the most widely used type. It is used when both articulating surfaces have been affected by disease and therefore is commonly used for osteoarthritis and rheumatoid arthritis.

Constrained TSA

Constrained designs involved the glenoid and humeral components coupled together and then fixed to the respective bone. They were originally designed for patients with an irreparable rotator cuff but the long-term results were not good (Neer, 1990). This design has now been superceded by the unconstrained type and is very rarely used.

Hemi-arthroplasty

The humeral head is replaced with a stemmed intramedullary implant that articulates with an unaffected and normal glenoid cavity. Thus these are used for severe fractures to the humeral head where no damage has occurred to the glenoid, and in rare cases of proximal humeral tumours.

Bipolar arthroplasty

Replacement of only the humeral surface but the humeral prosthesis has two articulations.

Hospital requirements

Most patients are admitted on the day of surgery and will stay in hospital for 3–5 days post-operatively. Standard pre-operative investigations such as routine blood tests, CXR and ECG are performed when indicated. Blood transfusion is unlikely and therefore donation of autologous blood is not required.

Radiology

Plain radiographs are taken to diagnose and plan the surgical procedure. Bone deficiency is best imaged with CT. The rotator cuff is best imaged with ultrasound or MRI.

Surgical anatomy and treatment

The surgery is performed with the patient in a supine position under general anaesthetic. The surgical approach most commonly used for shoulder arthroplasty is a deltopectoral incision (Fig. 8.4). This is a muscle interval between the deltoid and pectoralis major muscle that does not require detachment of these muscles. The short head of biceps brachii and coracobrachialis are retracted medially and the subscapularis muscle is identified. The subscapularis and anterior shoulder capsule are divided to

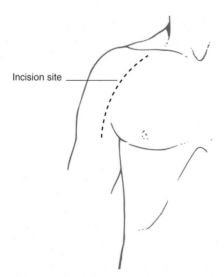

Incision site

Figure 8.4. Deltopectoral approach for total shoulder arthroplasty.

gain access to the shoulder joint and repaired at the end of the procedure. The other rotator cuff muscles are not detached (supraspinatus, infraspinatus and teres minor) unless the surgery is performed for fracture when these muscles are usually attached to the tuberosity fragments.

The arthritic or fractured portion of the humeral head is removed and the canal prepared to fit an intramedullary humeral component with a head the same size as that removed. The humeral component is placed in 20° of retroversion. The glenoid is then assessed and replaced if required. The muscles are repaired if divided and the wound closed over one drain.

Physiotherapy

Pre- and post-operative rehabilitation is very important in achieving a good outcome following shoulder arthroplasty. Pre-operative planning and education with patients prior to surgery is essential. The patient must understand that they will gain a significant reduction in pain following the procedure but that to expect full range of motion is unrealistic. Most patients can be expected to achieve a maximum of 120° elevation. Therefore the ability to resume certain functional overhead activities may not be possible following surgery.

Post-operative rehabilitation following a shoulder arthroplasty can vary between surgeon and patient. Neer (1990) classified patients into three groups: those with an intact rotator cuff, those in which the rotator cuff was repaired (active-assisted out to 6 weeks) and those with an irreparable and permanently damaged rotator cuff. Each group will require modification to their post-operative rehabilitation and goals. It is therefore vitally important that the physiotherapist communicates with the surgeon following the procedure to determine if the post-operative rehabilitation is to be limited in any way. As Neer (1990) states 'only the surgeon who performed the procedure should plan the schedule of exercises because only he/she knows the true pathology and strength of any repair'.

Generally the acute care rehabilitation protocol should consist of:

- DB&C
- F&A
- Passive or passive-assisted exercises with external rotation limited to neutral to allow subscapularis to heal.
- Hand and elbow exercises.
- Scapular retraction and depression exercises.
- Pendular exercises in or out of the sling.
- Resisted static contractions may commence at this stage but will depend on whether the rotator cuff was repaired. If the rotator cuff was intact then resisted static contractions of abduction, external rotation and flexion within pain limits can be commenced. If repaired, then resisted abduction, external and internal rotation should be avoided until the surgeon is confident that the repair can tolerate some simple strengthening exercises.
- Active exercises can be commenced as soon as the repaired tissue tolerates. This generally starts 2 weeks post-operatively and will

require the patient to attend out-patient physiotherapy. At this stage active flexion, internal rotation and external rotation and advanced muscle strengthening and stretching can be commenced.

Complications

Long-term follow-up of patients following shoulder replacement suggests that glenoid loosening is common and radiolucent lines are frequently observed at the cement-bone interface. Humeral loosening is not common. The incidence of glenoid loosening appears to be higher in patients with rotator cuff tears (Figgie et al., 1992). Instability and dislocation may be related to retroversion greater than 20°, a weak subscapularis repair, poor deltoid and rotator cuff function and glenoid bone defects. Other complications include rotator cuff tears, peri-prosthetic fractures, infection and neurovascular injury.

Shoulder instability

Patients presenting with acute anterior dislocation of the shoulder are normally treated with a closed reduction and conservative management. Closed reduction or relocation of the joint is often performed in the Emergency Department. This should be performed after a thorough neurological examination and exclusion of associated fractures and soft tissue damage. Most patients presenting to the Emergency Department with an acute dislocation are therefore not admitted to hospital and do not require further surgery. The exception is an acute dislocation in a young elite-level athlete. This is because the recurrence rate is high for these patients with non-operative management. A small percentage of patients may require immediate arthroscopic or open evaluation of the shoulder to assess and treat any associated damage. For instance, a Bankart lesion, which is detachment of the anterior labrum from the glenoid occurring due to the dislocation, may benefit from immediate repair.

Most commonly patients with symptomatic recurrent dislocation are those that may require elective surgery. Surgery may be required after a period of conservative management that has failed to prevent recurrent dislocations. In these cases the procedure is booked as an elective admission.

Recurrent dislocation has been separated into two main groups (Matsen et al. 1998). **T**raumatic **U**nidirectional associated with a **B**ankart lesion requiring **S**urgery (TUBS) and **A**traumatic **M**ultidirectional often **B**ilateral most requiring **R**ehabilitation and if requires surgery, then treated with an **I**nferior capsular shift (AMBRI).

Hospital requirements

Most arthroscopic procedures are performed as day surgery or an overnight stay, if there is inadequate pain control. Open procedures usually require an overnight stay in hospital.

Radiology

Plain radiographs including an A-P, lateral and axillary view of the shoulder will demonstrate dislocation or enlocation of the shoulder joint, glenoid rim fractures, Hill–Sach lesion and fractures of the greater tuberosity. CT arthrogram and MRI may provide further information on the integrity of intra-articular structures of the shoulder.

Surgical anatomy and treatment

The shoulder allows for great multi-direction range of motion and is an inherently unstable joint. Stability is maintained by multiple mechanisms that come into play at different positions of motion and applied forces. These include joint congruency that is enhanced by the glenoid labrum, negative intra-articular pressure within the joint, the shoulder capsule, the glenohumeral ligaments and the dynamic effects of the rotator cuff muscles and the biceps muscle.

Surgical treatment is directed to repairing or reconstructing all the pathology, including the Bankart lesion, capsular redundancy and other intra-articular pathology. Open or arthroscopic techniques can be used to repair the Bankart lesion. However in general, open procedures are required to successfully tighten the inferior capsule and glenohumeral ligaments. Recurrence rates are reported to be between 5–10 per cent for open techniques and 5–20 per cent for arthroscopic techniques. Benefits of arthroscopic stabilization again include a reduction of operative time, preservation of subscapularis, and less blood loss (Higgins and Warner, 2000). Although there are not as many long-term results of arthroscopic techniques, ideal patients are those that have a Bankart lesion with no significant capsular insufficiency and no other intra-articular pathology (Cole and Warner, 2000).

There are a variety of techniques for stabilizing the shoulder. Originally surgical techniques were designed to restore stability by compensating for the insufficiency in static restraints by a muscle or bony transfer. Techniques such as the Putti-Platt procedure (tightening and re-aligning the anterior capsule and subscapularis) and the Bristow procedure (transfer of the tip of the coracoid with its tendon attachments to the neck of the glenoid providing a bony block to dislocation) are rarely used except for revision procedures. Less invasive techniques that restore the static restraint to anterior translation are now more common.

Two of the more common techniques performed include the Bankart procedure and the inferior capsular shift. Both procedures can be performed via an open or arthroscopic approach.

Bankart procedure

The Bankart procedure involves opening the joint and incising the subscapularis muscle 3 cm from its insertion. This exposes the anterior capsule. The damaged capsule, along with any periosteum and labrum that has been avulsed, is sutured back onto the glenoid rim via drill holes, using devices such as bio-absorbable tacks. Subscapularis is then re-attached without any overlapping or shortening. This procedure is generally used for those patients with a traumatic unidirectional instability (TUBS).

Inferior capsular shift

The inferior capsular shift involves either splitting or incising through subscapularis and then through the capsule. The capsule is removed from the glenoid margin creating two flaps. The lower flap is raised and sutured higher on the glenoid rim and the upper flap is attached over the top of this. This essentially tightens the anterior shoulder capsule. The subscapularis splitting approach results in less deficit of external rotation due to the subscapularis muscle not being detached. This type of procedure is used for patients displaying multi-directional atraumatic instability (AMBRI).

Complications

Wound healing, infection and neurovascular injury rarely occur following these procedures. Recurrent dislocation may occur and depends on the pathology, operative technique, activity and age of the patient.

A functional restriction of external rotation may occur after anterior capsular repairs with non-anatomic repair of the subscapularis muscle and scar formation. However any stiffness is usually only limited to this range and it is not common for the stiffness to be global.

Physiotherapy

Following reconstructive surgery, the post-operative protocol usually requires that the patient wear a sling for 4–6 weeks. Obviously if subscapularis has been detached, shortened and re-attached then it is important that the post-operative protocol does not stretch or tighten this muscle.

Post-operative physiotherapy exercises should include:

- Shoulder retraction and depression exercises.
- Hand and wrist exercises.
- Strengthening exercises. Resisted static contractions of shoulder abduction, external rotation, adduction, extension and flexion can be performed. However, resisted static internal rotation should be avoided if the subscapularis was detached and sutured back.
- Pendular exercises in and out of the sling.
- Auto-assisted flexion can be performed within the patient's pain limits. Passive external rotation to neutral can be performed but the patient should not go beyond this position if subscapularis was detached and resutured.

Out-patient physiotherapy will be required to gradually increase the strength and movement in the shoulder. Patients should be seen 2 weeks post-operatively.

Manipulation under anaesthetic

Manipulation under anaesthetic (MUA) is usually reserved for patients with recalcitrant adhesive capsulitis. Adhesive capsulitis is primarily an inflammatory reaction in the capsule of the glenohumeral joint. The inflammation subsequently leads to formation of adhesions, specifically in the axillary fold and in the attachment of the capsule at the anatomic neck, causing severe restrictions in range of movement of the glenohumeral joint. This condition occurs more commonly in females in the 40 to 60 age group. This inflammation, with subsequent adhesion formation, may be primary (occurs for no known reason) or secondary to a period of immobilization. A period of immobilization may follow a fracture or other surgery around the chest and shoulder, such as a radical mastectomy.

The mainstay of treatment for this condition is conservative management including physiotherapy, analgesia, NSAIDs, local anaesthetic and steroid injections. Most patients should respond to this treatment or improve over time as the condition appears to resolve spontaneously within 18 months. However there may be some cases that do not respond to conservative treatment or the patient has functional requirements that must be addressed. In these cases, a MUA may be performed.

Technique

The manipulation is performed under general anaesthetic and a brachial plexus block may be used for post-operative pain relief. The technique involves abduction of the humerus with the scapula stabilized. To achieve this, the upper arm is held by the surgeon near to the shoulder to utilize a short lever arm. This breaks the inferior recess adhesions. The arm is then externally rotated and then internally rotated. It is common to hear the adhesions breaking and it is important not to use too much force or a long lever arm to prevent the humerus from breaking. The range of motion achieved under anaesthetic should be recorded and act as a guide for post-operative rehabilitation and patient expectations.

Open surgery is rarely required but may involve arthroscopic or open release of the contracted intra-articular structures. This is complex surgery as the space available for the arthroscope and operating instruments inside the joint is reduced. The complications are therefore higher than normal shoulder arthroscopy.

Physiotherapy

Physiotherapy is a prime consideration following MUA. If the adhesions are released then range of movement exercises must be instigated as soon as possible. In these cases, the physiotherapist should work very closely with the operating surgeon. It is often beneficial for the physiotherapist to observe the range of motion achieved in theatre. Immediately following the MUA, the physiotherapist can start passive and active range of motion. If necessary this may be performed in the recovery ward.

Active and passive elevation, abduction and external rotation should be performed. Ice or narcotic pain relief should be given prior to physiotherapy sessions.

Patients should be discharged with an exercise programme that mobilizes and stretches the operated shoulder to maintain and improve the range that was achieved in surgery.

Exercises following shoulder surgery

Wrist and hand exercises (Fig. 8.5)

Starting position

In standing with sling off. Maintain shoulder position by keeping the arm at the side.

Instruction

Bend the wrist first forwards then backwards. Rotate the wrist around in a circle. Make a fist then stretch the fingers out as straight as possible.

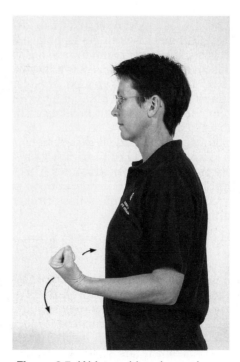

Figure 8.5. Wrist and hand exercises.

Elbow exercises (Fig. 8.6)

Starting position

In standing with sling off and maintaining the shoulder by the side.

Instruction

Bend your elbow fully then straighten as far as possible. Perform this first with the palm face directly up then with the palm facing down.

Scapular retraction and depression (Fig. 8.7)

Starting position

In standing or sitting.

Instruction

Keep the neck long and the chin tucked in. Pull the shoulder blades together and downwards. Hold for 10 seconds.

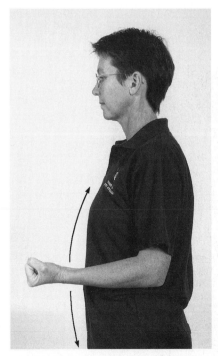
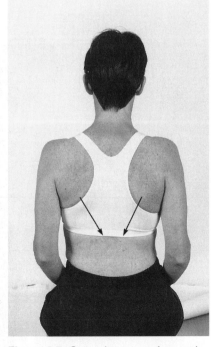

Figure 8.6. Elbow flexion and extension.

Figure 8.7. Scapular retraction and depression.

Pendular exercises

Starting position

Leaning over a secure table supported with the good arm leaning on the table. The arm can be either kept in the sling or taken out and elbow extended depending on the surgical procedure and amount of pain (Figs 8.8 and 8.9).

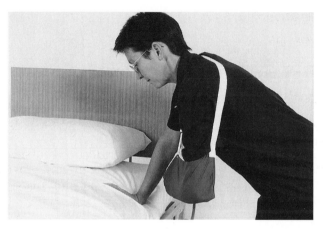

Figure 8.8. Pendular exercise in sling.

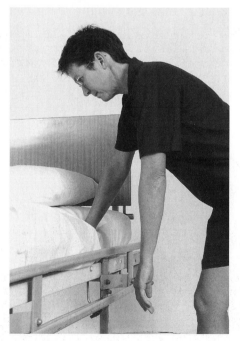

Figure 8.9. Pendular exercise with elbow extended.

Instruction

Gently let the arm rotate in a small circle, first clockwise then anti-clockwise.

Note: Gentle flexion/extension and abduction/adduction pendular exercises can be given but in the case of a rotator cuff repair, abduction should be avoided.

Passive elevation (Fig. 8.10)

Starting position

In supine lying, one pillow.

Instruction

With the elbow bent to a right angle, the physiotherapist or patient slowly lifts the affected arm as far as pain allows.

Note: This exercise can be progressed by gradually increasing the position to one of half-lying and then sitting. Thus gravity provides some additional resistance. The above exercise can also be progressed to an auto-assisted movement by having the elbow extended or asking the patient to hold onto a walking stick and lift through elevation (Fig. 8.11).

Resisted static shoulder exercises

Resisted static exercises should be performed after any shoulder surgery to maintain the muscle strength in the surrounding muscle. As previously discussed, some movements need to be avoided depending on the surgical procedure and muscular repair or re-attachment.

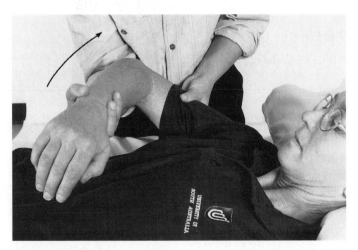

Figure 8.10. Passive elevation.

(a)

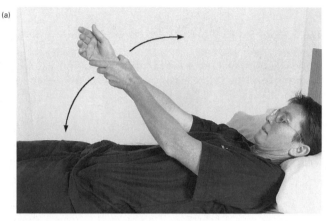

(b)

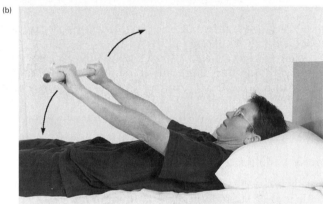

Figure 8.11. (a) Auto-assisted elevation. (b) Auto-assisted using a stick.

Starting position

Sitting with the arm by the side and elbow flexed to a right angle.

Instruction

Place the good hand on the inner aspect of the operated arm at the forearm. Gently try to push the wrist across the body but apply resistance with the non-operated hand. Do not allow the affected arm to move. This should be a hold only. Do not push through pain.

Note: The above exercise can be modified to provide resistance into abduction, external rotation, adduction, extension and flexion (Fig. 8.12a, b, c).

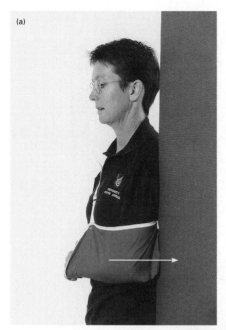
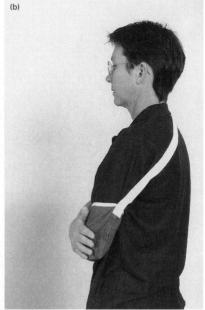
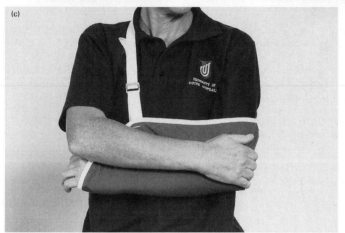

Figure 8.12. (a) Resisted extension against the frame of a door. (b) Self-resisted flexion. (c) Self-resisted abduction.

Mobilizing exercises

Pulley exercises (Fig. 8.13)

Position
Sitting or standing comfortably underneath the pulley.

Instruction
Use the good arm to slowly lift the affected arm through range.

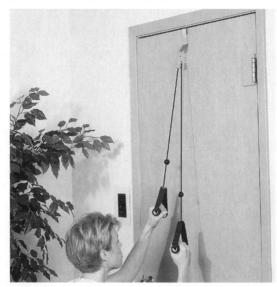

Figure 8.13. Auto-assisted elevation using a pulley (reproduced with permission from Smith and Nephew).

Note: Following a MUA patients must be advised to push through the limits of their pain whilst in other procedures pain may be the limiting factor.

External and internal rotation (Fig. 8.14)

Position
In supine lying with the elbows flexed to 90° whilst holding a light stick.

Instruction
Use the good arm to slowly rotate the affected arm away from and then across the body.

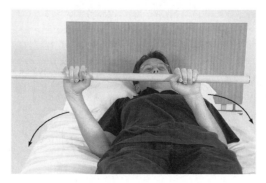

Figure 8.14. Auto-assisted external and internal rotation.

References

Altchek, D. W. (1995). Arthroscopy of the shoulder. *Scand. J. Med. Sci. Sports*, **5**, 71–75.

Ayub, E. (1991). Posture and the upper quarter. In *Physical Therapy of the Shoulder* (R. A. Donatelli, ed.), Churchill Livingstone.

Boileau, P. and Walch, G. (1997). Neer shoulder prosthesis results related to the etiology. In *Recent Advances in Upper Extremity Arthroplasty* (F. Schuind and K. N. An, eds.), World Scientific.

Bruzga, B. and Speer, K. (1999). Challenges of rehabilitation after shoulder surgery. *Clinics in Sports Med.*, **18**, 769–793.

Cole, B. J. and Warner, J. J. (2000). Arthroscopic versus open Bankart repair for traumatic anterior shoulder instability. *Clinics in Sports Med.*, **19**, 19–48.

Ellman, H., Hanker, G. and Bayer, M. (1986). Repair of the rotator cuff: end results of factors influencing reconstruction. *J. Bone Joint Surg.*, **68A**, 1136–1145.

Esch, J. C., Ozerkis, L. R., Helgager, J. A., Kane, N. et al. (1988). Arthroscopic subacromial decompression: results according to the degree of rotator cuff tear. *J. Arthroscop. Rel. Surg.*, **4**, 241–249.

Figgie, M. P., Inglis, A. E., Figgie, H. E., Sobel, M. et al. (1992). Custom total shoulder arthroplasty in inflammatory arthritis. *J. Arthroplasty*, **7**, 16.

Harryman, D. T., II, Mack, L. A., Wang, K. Y., Jackins, S. E., Richardson, M. L. and Matsen, F. A. (1991). Repairs of the rotator cuff: correlation of functional results with integrity of the cuff. *J. Bone Joint Surg.*, **73**, 982–989.

Hawkins, R. J., Bell, R. H. and Jallay, B. (1989). Total shoulder arthroplasty. *Clin. Orthop.*, **242**, 188–194.

Higgins, L. D. and Warner, J. J. (2000). Arthroscopic Bankart repair operative technique and surgical pitfalls. *Clinics in Sports Med.*, **19**, 49–62.

Jobe, F. W., Tibone, J. E., Jobe, C. E. and Kvitne, R. S. (1990). The shoulder in sports. In *The Shoulder* (C. A. Rockwood and F. A. Matsen, eds.) Vol. 2, WB Saunders Company.

Lazarus, M. D., Chansky, H. A., Misra, S., Williams, G. R. and Iannotti, J. P. (1994). Comparison of open and arthroscopic subacromial decompression. *J. Shoulder Elbow Surg.*, **3**, 1–11.

Liu, S. H. and Baker, C. L. (1994). Arthroscopically assisted rotator cuff repair: correlation of functional results with integrity of the cuff. *J. Arthroscop. Rel. Surg.*, **10**, 54–60.

Matsen, F. A. and Arntz, C. T. (1990). Subacromial impingement. In *The Shoulder* (C. A. Rockwood and F. A. Matsen, eds.) Vol. 2, pp. 623–636, WB Saunders Company.

Matsen, F. A., Thomas, S. C., Rockwood, C. A. and Wirth, M. A. (1998). Glenohumeral Instability. In *The Shoulder* (C. A. Rockwood and F. A. Matsen, eds.) Vol. 2 pp. 611–754, WB Saunders Company.

McConnell, J. (1991). A different approach to the assessment and treatment of shoulders. *Proceedings of the Upper Body Symposium – Cervical, Thoracic and Arm Pain*. Warnabool, Australia.

Neer, C. S. (1972). Anterior acromioplasty for the chronic impingement syndrome in the shoulder: a preliminary report. *J. Bone Joint Surg.*, **54A**, 41–50.

Neer, C. S. II (1983). Impingement lesions. *Clin. Orthop.*, **173**, 70–77.

Neer, C. S. (1990). *Shoulder Reconstruction*. pp. 143–269, WB Saunders Company.

Neer, C. S. II, Watson, K. C. and Stanton, F. J. (1982). Recent experiences in total shoulder replacement. *J. Bone Joint Surg.*, **64A**, 319–337.

Sachs, R. A., Stone, M. L. and Devine, S. (1994). Open vs. arthroscopic acromioplasty: a prospective, randomized study. *Arthroscopy*, **10**, 248–254.

Speer, K. P., Horowitz, L. and Warren, R. F. (1996). The efficacy of cryotherapy in the post-operative shoulder. *J. Shoulder Elbow Surg.*, **5**, 62–68.

Wilk, K. E., Harrelson, G. L., Arrigo, C. and Chmielewski, T. (1991). Shoulder Rehabilitation. In *Physical Rehabilitation of the Injured Athlete* (J. R. Andrews, G. L. Harrelson and K. E. Wilk, eds.) 2nd Edition, pp. 478–553, WB Saunders Company.

Wolfgang, G. L. (1974). Surgical repair of tears of the rotator cuff of the shoulder. *J. Bone Joint Surg.*, **56A**, 14–26.

CHAPTER 9

Surgery of the foot and ankle

The most common elective surgical procedures include correction of hallux valgus deformity, straightening of lesser toe deformities and arthrodesis of various joints of the foot and ankle. Patients presenting for these types of surgery often have co-existing medical conditions, such as rheumatoid arthritis, diabetes and peripheral vascular disease. These factors need to be assessed and considered prior to surgery and when planning the post-operative rehabilitation as they may affect wound healing, infection, recovery and mobilization following surgery. Emergency admissions generally include patients sustaining fractures or dislocations of the lower leg. These predominantly occur following high velocity trauma and commonly have significant soft tissue damage.

Hallux valgus

This deformity is characterized by a valgus and rotational deformity of the great toe at the level of the metatarsal-phalangeal (MTP) joint and in some cases may be associated with varus deformity of the 1st metatarsal (metatarsus primus varus). There is swelling at the level of the MTP joint due to bursal thickening and overgrowth of bone (exostosis).

This common condition has a genetic tendency that is further contributed to by inappropriate shoe wearing and is rarely seen in cultures that do not wear shoes. Hallux valgus is usually idiopathic but other causes to be considered include deformity secondary to contracture of the Achilles tendon, generalized ligamentous laxity, hypermobile 1st metatarsal joint, and spastic deformity from cerebral palsy and stroke.

The deformity is described by measuring two angles from standing plain radiographs. The hallux valgus angle (HV) is the angle between 1st metatarsal and the 1st proximal phalanx. The normal angle is less than 15° and represents the valgus shape of the MTP joint. The 1st–2nd intermetatarsal angle (1–2 MT) is the angle between the 1st and 2nd metatarsals. The normal value is less than 9° and represents the varus shape of the 1st metatarsal. A mild deformity is defined as a HV angle less than 20° and a 1–2 MT angle less than 11°. A severe deformity is defined as a HV angle greater than 40° and a 1–2 MT angle of greater than 16°.

There are many techniques that have been described to correct hallux valgus (Richardson, 1992a). In general they can be divided into distal soft tissue procedures, distal metatarsal osteotomies, proximal metatarsal osteotomies and medial procedures to remove the exostosis and capsular plications. Most mild deformities are corrected with an osteotomy of the distal metatarsal, removal of exostosis and medial capsular plication. More severe deformities require a distal release of the contracted tissues of the MTP joint to correct the valgus and rotational deformity of the hallux and a proximal metatarsal osteotomy to correct the varus deformity of the metatarsal. Internal fixation with K-wires is commonly used to hold the correction until the osteotomy has united.

In general, the post-operative management of hallux valgus and other fore-foot procedures consists of a firm fore-foot dressing applied for 2 weeks. The wounds are checked at this stage and a dressing reapplied for a further 4 weeks. Patients are allowed to weight bear as tolerated in a rigid soled shoe. Small Kirschner wires (K-wires) that have been used to hold the bones and joints in position during the initial healing are removed in the out-patient clinic at 46 weeks after insertion (Fig. 9.1).

The most common complications include wound healing problems and infection. Minor discharge and redness around the pin sites is not uncommon and usually settles with regular dressings and oral antibiotic medication. Removal of the wires may be indicated if this progresses to local infection. It is important to inform the patients that 40 per cent of patients will not fit into the shoes of their choice after surgery, despite having a narrower foot and good surgical correction.

Lesser toe deformities

Claw toes are characterized by flexion of the interphalangeal (IP) joints and hyperextension of the MTP joints. This may be due to neurological

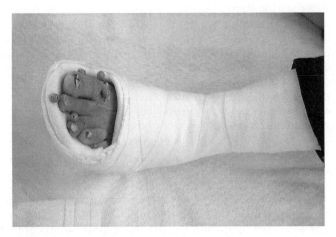

Figure 9.1. Below knee cast with K-wires.

disorders and these should be excluded. The deformity is initially flexible but later becomes fixed and the MTP joints may then subluxate or dislocate resulting in callosities under the metatarsal heads or over the IP joints.

Hammer toes are characterized by proximal interphalangeal (PIP) joint flexion, MTP and distal interphalangeal extension or hyperextension. The second toe of one or both feet are most commonly affected and this is often caused by long toes in short shoes. The MTP joints may subluxate or dislocate and callosities may develop under the metatarsal heads or over the IP joints.

Mallet toes are a flexion deformity of the distal interphalangeal (DIP) joint with initially normal PIP and MTP joints.

Deformities of the lesser toes usually result in painful callosities due to abnormal loading and subluxation or dislocation of the metatarsal heads and pressure over the dorsum of the IP joints from poorly fitted shoewear. Deformities are either flexible and correctable or fixed and rigid. Flexible deformities can be corrected with tendon releases and transfers. Fixed deformity requires joint release, excision arthroplasty or arthrodesis. Temporary K-wire fixation may be performed to place the toes in a straight position after surgery. A fore-foot dressing is applied and the patients can mobilize as tolerated (Richardson, 1992b).

Ankle arthrodesis

Ankle arthrodesis is indicated for the treatment of end-stage ankle arthrosis associated with pain and deformity and for the salvage of failed ankle replacement. Various techniques using internal or external fixation have been described to obtain fusion of the ankle joint. Most commonly a lateral approach is made and the distal fibula is excised to give access to the ankle joint and for use as local bone graft. Bone graft from the iliac crest is usually not required. The ankle is fused in a position of neutral dorsiflexion, 5° of hind-foot valgus and 5–7° of fore-foot external rotation.

Post-operatively the patient is placed in a below knee back slab until the wounds have healed and swelling has subsided and then into a below knee cast. The patient is non-weight bearing for the first 6 weeks, and then is allowed to weight bear in the cast for a further 6 weeks or until union is seen on plain radiographs.

The common complications include wound healing and infection problems, malalignment due to incorrect positioning at the time of surgery and approximately a 5 per cent non-union rate.

Triple arthrodesis

A triple arthrodesis is a fusion of the three joints of the hind foot, namely the talo-navicular (TN), calcaneo-cuboid (CC) and subtalar joints. The operation is indicated for arthrosis of the subtalar and either one or both of the TN or CC joints, unstable subtalar and midtarsal joints due to neuromuscular disorders or hind-foot malalignment. Surgery is usually performed through two separate incisions, one lateral and one medial. The foot is placed in a plantigrade position (neutral dorsiflexion) with the subtalar joint in 3–5° valgus, the transverse tarsal joints in neutral adduction/abduction and the fore foot in neutral varus/valgus. Post-operatively the patient is placed in a below knee back slab until the wounds have healed and swelling has subsided then into a below knee cast. Patients are treated non-weight bearing for the first 6 weeks and then allowed to weight bear as tolerated in a cast for a further 6 weeks or until union.

Complications include wound healing and infection. Non-union is uncommon but if it does occur it is usually at the TN joint. Malalignment due to incorrect positioning at the time of surgery may prevent normal mobilization. In the long term, 30 per cent of patients will develop degenerative changes in the ankle joint.

Ankle fractures

Fractures around the ankle are commonly seen following twisting injuries at sport, motor vehicle accidents and low velocity falls in osteoporotic middle-aged women. Because of the lack of soft tissue in this region, open wounds, skin problems and neurovascular injury are not uncommon. The terminology of ankle fractures is based on three malleoli and fractures are often described as bi- or tri-malleolar. The medial and lateral malleoli are true anatomical structures representing the distal portion of the tibia and fibula; the posterior malleolus is used to describe the radiographic projection of the posterior part of the distal tibia.

There are many classification systems for ankle fractures. The Lauge–Hansen classification system is based on mechanism of injury but the Weber system (Types A, B and C) is most commonly used and helps explain the fracture type, associated injuries and assists in surgical planning. The AO system is an expansion of the Weber system and is often used for research. The Weber system refers to the lateral malleolus fracture only. The medial or posterior malleoli may or may not be fractured in each type but will provide information on the state of the syndesmosis between the tibia and fibula (Van der Griend et al., 1996).

Type A fracture is a transverse avulsion fracture of the fibula at or below the level of the ankle joint. The medial malleolus may be intact or sheared, and there may be an associated compression fracture of the tibial edge. The tibio-fibular ligament complex is always intact. Most can be treated in a plaster if minimally displaced or with minimal internal fixation.

Type B fracture is a spiral fracture of the distal fibula beginning at the level of the syndesmosis. Part of the tibio-fibular syndesmotic ligament may be involved but the ankle mortise is stable following reduction of the fracture. These fractures can be treated in a plaster if there is less than 3 mm displacement and no talar shift. Otherwise they are treated with open reduction and internal fixation using a plate and screws.

Type C fracture is a fracture of the fibula anywhere between the syndesmosis and the head of the fibula. The tibio-fibular ligament complex is always disrupted and in most cases a diastasis screw should be inserted if the syndesmosis remains unstable after fixation of the fracture with open reduction and internal fixation.

Complications of fractures around the ankle include wound healing and infection problems, non-union and degenerative arthritis if the fracture has not been reduced anatomically.

Calcaneal fractures

The calcaneum is the most commonly fractured bone of the foot, accounting for approximately 60 per cent of tarsal fractures and 2 per cent of all fractures. The mechanism is a fall from a height in 80–90 per cent of patients. Ten per cent of calcaneal fractures are associated with lumbar spine fractures. Five to 10 per cent are bilateral whilst one quarter of patients sustain associated lower limb injuries. Careful initial assessment for associated injuries is important when an isolated calcaneal fracture is diagnosed. Calcaneal fractures are classified as extra- or intra-articular and can be further described according to the number and location of the articular fragments based on CT scans.

There is a current trend for more aggressive treatment of these fractures with open reduction and internal fixation although the learning curve and complication rate is initially high (Sanders, 2000). Generally undisplaced, extra-articular fractures require conservative management. Intra-articular fractures, however, require surgery to restore the height, length and width of the calcaneum and to restore as close as normal joint surface alignment. Most procedures are performed through a curved lateral approach. Initially post-operative management involves rest in a back slab with the leg elevated until the swelling is reduced. Following this a below knee non-weight bearing cast for 6–12 weeks. Weight bearing is not allowed until 12 weeks.

Complications

Complications include the impingement of the peroneal nerves against the lateral malleolus. Calcaneal widening, varus and valgus deformities, reflex sympathetic dystrophy, chronic heel pad pain and post-traumatic arthritis of the subtalar joint can also occur.

Achilles tendon rupture

Complete rupture of the Achilles tendon occurs through a relatively hypovascular area of the tendon which is between 2–6 cm above the insertion into the calcaneus. The tendon has been shown to degenerate due to repetitive microtrauma over a period of time in some patients although the majority are asymptomatic prior to the injury. However, the final rupture occurs during either forced dorsiflexion against a contracted heel cord or in sudden acceleration. Simmond's test is diagnostic and is performed with the patient prone, passive squeezing of the calf fails to plantar-flex the foot (may also be called Thompson's test). Ultrasound or MRI will demonstrate a tear if clinically in doubt.

Treatment of acute ruptures will differ between surgeons. There is no significant functional difference between operative and non-operative management if the tendon heals. The re-rupture rate has been reported to be between 2–7 per cent for operative management and between 8–35 per cent for conservative non-operative management. Late repair of a chronic rupture requires a more complex operative management and possible tendon graft. Conservative and operative management require cast immobilization for 8 weeks. Some surgeons favour early protected weight bearing in a splint after surgical repair.

Complications of Achilles tendon repair include re-rupture, tendon adhesions and stiffness of ankle with reduced dorsiflexion. Operative treatment is also associated with a small incidence of wound healing, infection and neuroma problems, which do not occur with non-operative management.

Physiotherapy

In-patient physiotherapy management following surgery to the ankle or foot will involve the principles of management discussed in Chapters 3 and 4. All patients should receive immediate post-operative prophylactic exercises including deep respiratory and foot and ankle exercises. Most patients will be required to have a lower leg plaster cast, dressing or splint. The physiotherapist must educate each patient on the care and use of any cast or dressing, with emphasis on noting for compartment syndrome or cast tightness.

Specific exercise prescription should include mobilizing exercises to the joints above and below the cast or dressing to prevent stiffness in the unaffected joints. Thus in a lower leg cast, knee extension and flexion exercises should be prescribed. Resisted static exercises of the muscles within the cast should also be given. However, note should be made of the operating procedure as in some cases muscle action may be contra-indicated, e.g. immediately following Achilles tendon repair.

Gait training and weight-bearing status will depend on the surgical procedure and requirements of the surgeon. Patients must be taught how to effectively and safely manage assistive devices so that they are functionally independent.

References

Richardson, E. G. (1992a). Disorders of the hallux. In *Campbell's Operative Orthopaedics* (A. H. Crenshaw, ed.) 8th Edition, pp. 2615–2692, CV Mosby Co.

Richardson, E. G. (1992b). Lesser toe abnormalities. In *Campbell's Operative Orthopaedics* (A. H. Crenshaw, ed.) 8th Edition, pp. 2729–2755, CV Mosby Co.

Sanders, R. (2000). Current concepts review – displaced intra-articular fractures of the calcaneus. *J. Bone Joint Surg.*, **82A**, 225–250.
Van der Griend, R., Michelson, J. D. and Bone, L. B. (1996). Instructional course lectures –
fractures of the ankle and the distal part of the tibia. *J. Bone Joint Surg.*, **78A**, 1772–1783.

Index

Achilles tendon rupture, 150
Acromioplasty, 1227
Adult respiratory distress
    syndrome, *see* Fat embolism
Analgesia
    epidural, 85
    patient controlled, 30, 85
Analgesics, 30
Anatomy
    bone, 1
    cartilage, 3
    femoral head blood supply, 95
    ligaments, 2
    meniscus, 2
    tendons, 2
Ankle
    arthrodesis, 148
    fractures, 149
Anterior cruciate ligament
Antibiotics, 34
Anticoagulant drugs, 32
AO classification of fractures, 12,
    149
Arthrodesis
    ankle, 148
    triple, 148
    shoulder 131
Arthroscopic
    acromioplasty, 127
    reconstruction of anterior
        cruciate ligament, 114
Arthroscopy
    hip, 97
    knee, 109

    shoulder, 127
Aspirin for DVT prophylaxis, 33
Assessment for physiotherapy, 35
Atelectasis prevention of, 39
Austin-Moore prosthesis, 93
Avascular necrosis
    femoral head, 95, 97
    pathology, 5
Axonotmesis from fractures, 22

Bankart
    lesion, 134
    procedure, 135
Bed rest prolonged, mobilization
        after, 58
Blood transfusion autologous, 28
Bone
    anatomy, 1
    graft and screws, 18
Breathing exercises, 39, 40
Bristow procedure, 135

Calcaneocuboid joint, 148
Calcaneum fracture, 150
Callus, 12
Capsulitis adhesive, 128, 137
Care map, 45, 46
Cartilage
    anatomy, 3
    degeneration grades 1–4, 4
    injury, 3
Casts, 15

Charnley abduction pillow, 85
Chest exercises, 39
Chondroplasty, 109
Collagen types, 2
Compartment syndrome, 24
Compression
  hip screw, 95
  screw plate, 19
Continuous passive motion, 116
  device, 106
Critical pathway, 45
Cruciate ligament reconstruction,
  113, 114
  complications, 117
Crutches, 52, 55, 56
Cryocuff
  for pain relief, 107
  for shoulder, 128

Deep vein thrombosis prevention,
  41, 43
  physiotherapy, 44
Discharge documents, 48
Dislocation
  hip, 84, 90
  shoulder 134
Documentation importance of, 36
Draw sheet for moving patients,
  73
Driving after hip replacement, 89
Dual energy X-ray absorptiometry,
  5
DVT, *see* Deep vein thrombosis
Dynamic
  compression plates, 13
  hip screw, 19

Edinburgh collar and cuff, 128
Enoxaparin, 32
Exercise
  closed kinetic chain, 113, 116
  open chain kinetic, 113, 116
Exercises
  after ankle operations, 151
  after hip operations, 97, 98
  after hip replacement, 85
  after knee arthroscopy, 112

after repair of shoulder
  dislocation, 136
after shoulder operations, 129,
  138
after shoulder arthroplasty, 133
breathing and coughing, 39, 40
elbow, 139
foot and ankle
  after knee replacement, 107
  to prevent DVT, 44
pendular, 140
quadriceps, 107, 120
scapular, 139
walking, 51
wrist and hand, 138
External fixation, 20

Fasciotomy for compartment
  syndrome, 25
Fat embolism, 23
Fibula fracture, 149
Fixation
  external 20
  internal, 17
Fluid intravenous, 28
Foot surgery, 146
Fracture
  ankle, 149
  avulsion, 8
  calcaneum, 150
  classification, 9
    AO system, 12
  complications
    compartment syndrome, 24
    damage to surrounding
      structures, 22
    haemorrhage, 21
    wound infection, 22
  external fixation, 20
  greenstick, 11
  healing, 12
    factors affecting, 14
  immobilization, 15
  internal fixation, 17
  pathological, 7
  pathology, 6, 9
  proximal femur, 92
    epidemiology, 94
  reduction, 15

Fracture (*cont.*)
  stress, 7
  subcapital Garden classification,
    92
  treatment, 14
    internal fixation, 17
    splinting, 20
    traction, 17
Frames walking, 53

Gait, *see* Walking
Garden classification of proximal
    femoral fractures, 92

Hallux valgus, 146
Hamilton-Russell traction, 18
Healing tendons, 2
Healthcare workers injured by
    lifting, 66
Hemiarthroplasty, 93
Heparin, 32
Hip
  arthroscopy, 97
  arthroplasty, *see* replacement
  replacement, 78
    complications
      confusion, 90
      dislocation, 84, 90
      foot drop, 91
      leg length inequality, 91
      sciatic nerve damage, 91
    driving after, 89
    hospital requirements, 82
    indications, 81
    mobilization after, 87
    outcomes, 80
    revision, 84
    surgical anatomy, 83
    technique, 83
Hoists, hydraulic, 67, 76
Hypovolaemic shock, 22

Impingement syndrome in
    shoulder, 126
Intramedullary nail, 13, 18
Intravenous fluid, 28
Investigations medical, 26

Joint replacement
  complication infection, 23
  hip, 78
  knee, 102
  shoulder, 131

Kirschner wires for hallux valgus,
    147
Knee
  arthroscopy, 109, 111
    complications, 112
  medial collateral ligament
      injury, 114
  medial meniscus injury, 114
  replacement, 102
    complications, 108
    indications, 104
    physiotherapy after, 107
    surgical anatomy, 105
    technique, 105
    unicompartmental, 103

Labral tear, 97
Lachman test, 113
Lauge Hansen classification, 149
Lifting
  equipment, 76
  techniques, 66
Ligament
  anatomy, 2
  injuries, 2
  medial collateral of knee injury,
      114
Litigation fear of, 36
Log rolling, 68
Lung atelectasis, 39

Magnetic resonance imaging for
    knee lesions, 111
Manipulation under anaesthetic,
    137
Medication, 30
  analgesics, 30
  antibiotics, 34
  anticoagulant, 32
  anti-emetics, 33

Medication (*cont.*)
  gastro-intestinal protective
      agents, 34
  NSAIDs, 32
Meniscectomy, 110
Meniscus
  anatomy, 2
  medial injury, 114
  repair, 111
Mobilization
  after hip replacement, 87
  after prolonged bed rest, 58
  after proximal femoral fracture,
      96
  in bed 69
Monkey bar, 76
Moving patients, 66

Neurapraxia from fractures, 22
Neurotmesis from fractures, 22
Non-steroidal anti-inflammatory
      drugs, 32
Normal values, 27

Open reduction and internal
      fixation, 17
Osteoarthritis
  hip, 81
  pathology, 3
Osteonecrosis, *see* Avascular
      necrosis
Osteoplasty, 109
Osteoporosis
  causing femoral fracture, 94
  pathology, 5
Oxygen for treatment, 29

Pagets disease pathology, 6
Patella retinaculum release, 110
Patient controlled analgesia, 30, 85
Peroneal nerve palsy, 108
Pivot shift test, 113
Plate and screws, 18
Polymethylmethacrylate cement,
      78
Pre-admission clinic, 82

Preoperative physiotherapy
      education, 45
Pressure sores, 23
  prevention, 69
Problem-oriented medical record,
      36
Prophylactic physiotherapy, 38
Putti-Platt procedure, 135

Quadriceps exercises, 120

Ranitidine, 34
Records problem oriented, 36
Rehabilitation
  after cruciate ligament
      reconstruction, 115, 118
  after shoulder arthroplasty, 133
Rheumatoid arthritis pathology, 4
Rolling, 66, 71
Rotator cuff, 125
  tears, 127

Screw
  compression hip, 95
  plate compression, 19
  transfixion, 19
Shoulder
  arthroplasty, 131
  dislocation, 134
  exercises
      passive, 141
      pulley, 143
  frozen, 128
  lesions, 124
  lift, 74
  manipulation under anaesthetic,
      137
Simmond s test, 151
Sitting up, 72
Slings, 128
SOAP assessment, 35
  for hip replacement, 82
Splint, 20
  Zimmer 21
Stairs lessons in using, 61
Stick walking, 54

Stiffness after knee replacement, 109
Stride stance position, 74
Subacromial space, 124
Subtalar joint, 148

Talonavicular joint, 148
Tendo achilles, 150
Tendon
  anatomy, 2 *see also* Tendo achilles
  healing, 2
  rupture Achilles, 150
Thompson's test, 151
Thrombosis prevention, 41
Toe
  deformities, 147
  hammer, 148
  mallet, 148
Total
  hip replacement, *see* Hip replacement
  knee replacement, *see* Knee replacement
Transfer of patients, 67
Trauma, *see* Fracture, Dislocation
Trendelenburg gait, 84

Urinary catheter, 29

Vitamin C and fracture healing, 14

Walking
  aids, 52
  education after knee replacement, 108
  exercises, 51
  patterns, 57
  training, 60
    after hip replacement, 89
Warfarin, 32
Weber classification, 149
Weed's system, 36
Weight bearing
  after hip replacement, 87
  definitions, 51
Wire bands, 19
Wound infection from fractures, 22

Zimmer splint, 21